DIABETIC RENAL DIET COOKBOOK FOR BEGINNERS

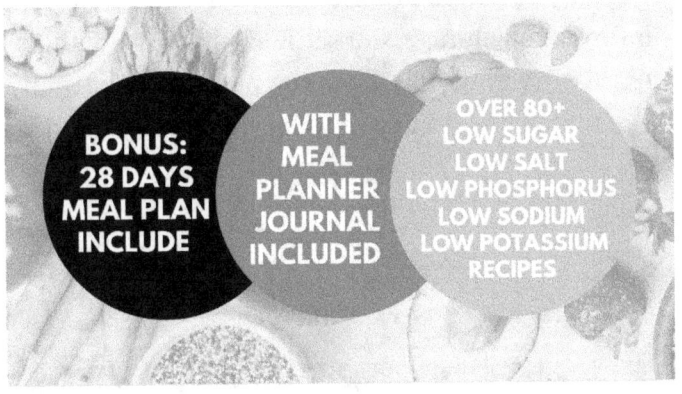

Tasty Easy To Make Low Sugar & Low Salt Recipes That Support Kidney Health And Slow Diabetes Progression For Optimum Health

Nancy K. Doctor

©Nancy K. Doctor

Copyright © 2024 by Nancy K. Doctor

All rights reserved.
No part of this book may be reproduced in any form or by any electronic or mechanical means, including information storage and retrieval systems, without permission in writing from the publisher, except by a reviewer who may quote brief passages in a review.

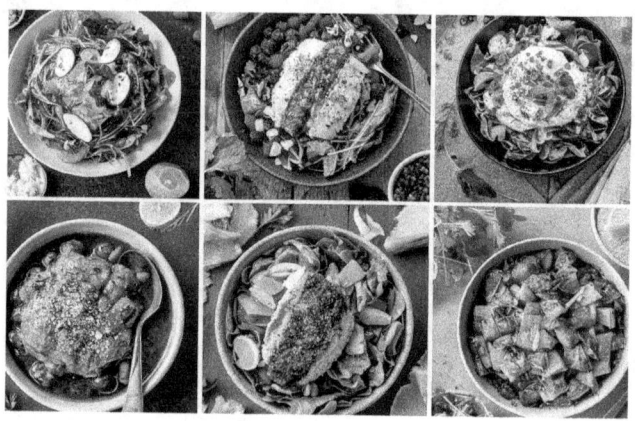

©Nancy K. Doctor

TABLE OF CONTENTS

INTRODUCTION.. 6
CHAPTER 1..8
DIABETES RENAL GROCERY LISTS................. 8
    Milk And Non-dairy Options....................... 8
    Breads And Starches................................. 9
    Fruits And Drinks......................................9
    Starchy Veggies...................................... 10
    Non-starchy Veggies............................... 11
    Meat, Cheese, And Eggs........................ 11
    Seasoning and Calories.......................... 12
    Beverages... 12
    Cold Cereals... 12
    Miscellaneous... 13
    Sweets.. 13
    5 Tips for Making a Diabetic Kidney Disease Diet Work for You... 14
CHAPTER 2...16
APPETIZERS AND BREAKFAST IDEAS............16
    Spicy Tofu Scrambler............................. 16
    Renal-Friendly Garden Veggie Frittata........... 17
    Cranberry Almond Bulgur Cereal................. 18
    Charred Red Bell Pepper Chickpea Spread... 20
    Tangy Asparagus Spears........................20
    Creamy Peanut Butter Chickpea Dip.............. 22
    Classic Chickpea Spread........................ 23
    Grilled Veggie Avocado Dip..................... 24
    Spinach and Mushroom Egg Cups.................. 25
    Oven-Baked Yogurt and Lemon Chicken Nuggets...26

©Nancy K. Doctor

Peanut Butter Infused Oatmeal Bliss.............. 28
BEVERAGE AND SMOOTHIES......................... **29**
   Refreshing Lime and Mint Tea....................... 29
   Refreshing Lime Mockarita.......................... 30
   Strawberry Lime Bliss................................ 31
PASTRY/DESSERT....................................**33**
   Savory Chicken Zucchini Pie....................... 33
   Nutritious Whole-Grain Soda Bread................34
   Mixed-Grain Raspberry Muffins..................... 36
   Warmly Spiced Carrot and Raisin Loaf........... 38
   Savory Southwestern Cornmeal Muffins.........40
   Wholesome Muesli Energy Bars.....................42
   Traditional Irish Whole-Wheat Bread.............. 44
   Berry Delight Whole-Grain Coffee Cake......... 45
   Rustic Apple-Cranberry Tart............................47
   Spiced Carrot Raisin Loaf............................... 49
   Wholesome Apple Pie.....................................51
MAIN DISH/LUNCH....................................**52**
   Seared Salmon with Braised Broccoli.............52
   Rosemary Infused Chicken Skewers.............. 55
   Oven-Baked Salmon with Asparagus on Whole-Grain Bun..56
   Couscous Stuffed Peppers........................... 57
   Low Sodium Stir Fry...59
   Nutritious Blueberry Whole-Wheat Pancakes. 61
   Ultimate Vegetable Stir-Fry............................. 62
   Sweet Potato Waffles with Homemade Blueberry Syrup.. 64
   Scalloped Corn-Stuffed Bell Peppers..............66
   Spinach and Mushroom Egg-Light Frittata..... 68

Smoky Bean and Mushroom Cornucopias..... 70
Spring Vegetable Rice Noodles...................... 72
Spinach, Chickpea, and Raisin Pasta............ 74
Tropical Mango Salsa Pizza............................76
Classic Hummus... 77
Grilled Pork Tenderloin Fajitas....................... 78
Zesty Fish Tacos with Tomatillo Salsa............80

SALAD..82

Herb-Infused French Lentil Salad................... 82
Apple, Cranberry, and Walnut Salad...............84
Tangy Pickled Onion and Herb Salad............. 85
Pear and Fennel Salad with Walnuts.............. 86
Chilled Shrimp and Apple Stuffed Tomatoes...88
Fresh Spinach and Mixed Berry Salad........... 90
Honey-Dressed Warm Cabbage and Carrot Slaw... 91
Tri-Color Tomato Basil Salad......................... 93

SAUCE AND DRESSING...96

Sweetened Balsamic Dressing....................... 96
Creamy Greek Yogurt Ranch Dressing...........97
Honeyed Peach Puree.................................... 99
Nutty Chickpea Spread................................. 100

SIDE DISHES... 102

Refreshing Sugar-Free Coleslaw.................. 102
Quick and Nutritious Tuna Salad.................. 103
Simple Cauliflower Rice................................ 104
Kale and Broccoli Power Bowl...................... 105
Sweet Honey and Sage Glazed Carrots....... 106
Easy Fried Rice..107
Savory Roasted Asparagus and Mushroom

- Medley Stew..109
- Strawberry Fruit Salad......................................110
- Cobb Salad with Dijon Dressing..........................111
- Quick Pickled Vegetables..................................113
- Flavourful Lean Country Sausage.......................114
- Golden Lemon Almond Rice..............................115
- Quick Roasted Green Beans..............................117
- Delicious Spiced Buckwheat Pilaf.......................118
- Nutritious Tangy Green Beans............................120
- Hearty Vegetable Barley and Mushroom Soup.....121

SNACKS...124
- Almond Essence Cookies.................................124
- Spicy Cream Cheese Tortilla Rolls......................125
- Almond-Infused Pear Parfait..............................127

DINNER RECIPES..128
- Gingered Cranberry Chicken Delight...................128
- Zesty Lemon Thyme Tuna Pasta Salad...............130
- Mexican-Inspired Turkey and Rice Stuffed Peppers...132
- Homemade Chicken Pad Thai...........................134

CONCLUSION..136

BONUS..138
- 28-Days Meal Plan...138
- MEAL PLANNER JOURNAL............................146
- Groceries Shopping List Planner........................154
- The Free Ebook Download................................162

©Nancy K. Doctor

INTRODUCTION

Living with chronic kidney disease (CKD) means your kidneys have to work overtime to clear out waste and toxins and excess fluids. When diabetes mixes, it becomes even trickier to manage your blood sugar levels and potentially leading to further damage in your kidneys blood vessels. Moreover diabetes have a knack for hiking up your blood pressure and contributing to additional strain on your kidneys. Shockingly 1 in 3 adults with diabetes also battles with CKD making the management of these conditions a hefty task. Yet embracing a diet tailored for both kidney disease and diabetes can be a game changer in regaining control. Proper nutrition is key to managing both ailments effectively. However, it is crucial to consult with your healthcare provider or a dietitian before making significant dietary changes.

Picture this: You are about to enjoy a meal that's not only delectable but also nourishes and a feast that delights your taste buds simultaneously boosts your well being. For those juggling diabetes and kidney disease, such a meal might seem like a distant fantasy and give the usual array of bland and restrictive diet options. But what if there's a different path?

I welcome you to a culinary revolution where every bit is a step toward mastering your health. The

©Nancy K. Doctor

"Diabetic Renal Diet Cookbook for Beginners" isn't just a collection of recipes; it is a passport to rediscovering the joy of eating while adeptly managing your health conditions.

I get it—the frustration of adhering to a strict diet that's low in sodium, potassium, sugar and salt can be overwhelming. It can feel like you're missing out on life's flavorful mosaic. But what if limitations could spark creativity? With the right guidance and ingredients, you can dive into a world of scrumptious and' wholesome meals tailored to your needs. This book aims to be your companion in that world.

Offering more than just recipes, this book provides a clear explanation of the complexities of diabetes and kidney disease along with irresistible recipes and straightforward instructions. It's a beacon of hope showing that within dietary limits, your life can still be vibrant and delicious. Through the power of food, you can lead a joyful and flavorful life.

So are you ready to uncover the tasty opportunities that await you? Flip the pages and embark on a culinary adventure that will transform your eating habits and empower you to reclaim your health and one delightful bite at a time.

©Nancy K. Doctor

CHAPTER 1

DIABETES RENAL GROCERY LISTS

Milk And Non-dairy Options

Recommended;
- Non-dairy creamer
- Plain yogurt
- Sugar-free yogurt
- Sugar-free pudding
- Sugar-free ice cream
- Sugar-free non-dairy frozen desserts

Due to their high protein, potassium, or phosphorus content, dairy products are frequently limited to 4-ounce portions.

Limit or Avoid;
- Cocoa-infused milk
- Cultured milk
- Flavored yogurts with added sugars
- Sweetened custards
- Frozen dairy desserts
- Sweetened non-dairy frozen confections

Breads And Starches

Recommended;
Whole grain, whole wheat, and white bread varieties, including rye and sourdough, as well as plain, unflavored dry cereals, semolina-based Cream of Wheat, hominy grits, Malt-O-Meal, and traditional oatmeal. Additionally, various pasta types such as white and whole wheat, along with diverse rice options like brown, white, and wild rice. Small-sized bagels, hamburger rolls, crackers without added salt, homemade cornbread, and tortillas crafted from wheat or corn flour also fall within this category.

limit or Avoid;
Bran bread, frosted or sugar-coated cereals, quick cereals, bran or granola, gingerbread, pancake mix, cornbread mix, biscuits, and salty snacks (such as potato chips, corn chips, and crackers). Whole wheat cereals, such as wheat flakes and raisin bran, as well as whole grain hot cereals, contain more phosphorus and potassium than refined ones, but may still be restricted.

Fruits And Drinks

Recommended;
Apples, apple juice, applesauce, apricot halves, berries such as

strawberries, raspberries, cranberries, blackberries, and blueberries, low sugar cranberry juice, cherries, fruit cocktail, grapefruit, grapes, grape juice, kumquats, mandarin oranges, pears, pineapple, plums, tangerine, watermelon, fruit canned in unsweetened juice.

Limit or Avoid;
avocados, bananas, cantaloupe, dried fruits (dates, raisins, prunes), honeydew melon, kiwis, Kumquats, mandarin oranges, pears, pineapple, plums, tangerines, watermelon, and fruit preserved in juice without added sugar.

Starchy Veggies

Recommended;
Opt for choices such as corn, peas, and blends containing these elements, though it is suggested to consume them sparingly due to their elevated phosphorus content. Additionally, if necessary, potatoes can be pre-soaked to reduce their potassium levels before consumption. Dried beans and peas may be included in restricted amounts, depending on your dietitian's recommendations.

Limit or Avoid;
Baked potatoes, sweet potatoes, yams, baked beans, succotash, pumpkin, and winter squash.

Non-starchy Veggies

Recommended;
Asparagus, beets, broccoli, Brussels sprouts, carrots, cabbage, cauliflower, celery, cucumber, eggplant, frozen broccoli slices, green beans, iceberg lettuce, kale, leeks, mustard greens, okra, onions, red and green peppers, radishes, raw spinach, snow peas, summer squash, and turnips.

Limit or Avoid;
Fresh artichokes, newly harvested bamboo sprouts, chard from beets, nopal cactus, steamed bok choy, cultivated kohlrabi, mashed swedes, fermented cabbage, wilted spinach, ripe tomatoes, concentrated tomato puree, and tomato liquid extract

Meat, Cheese, And Eggs

Recommended;
Lean cuts of meat, poultry, fish, and shellfish; eggs, low cholesterol egg alternative; natural cheeses (in restricted quantities) Cottage cheese (restricted owing to the high salt level)

Limit Or Avoid;
Bacon, canned and luncheon meats, processed cheese,

hot dogs, organ meats, almonds, pepperoni, salami, salmon and sausage

Seasoning and Calories

Recommended;
Low-fat mayonnaise, sour cream, and cream cheese, as well as soft or tub margarine,

Limit or avoid;
Bacon fat, back fat, butter, Crisco®, lard, shortening, margarines with trans fats, whipped cream

Beverages

Recommended;
Water, diet clear sodas, homemade tea, or lemonade flavored with a low-calorie sweetener.

lemonade containing sugar, syrup, or

Limit or Avoid;
Regular or diet dark colas, beer, fruit juices, fruit-flavored beverages, bottled or canned iced tea or phosphoric acid; sugar-sweetened tea or lemonade

Cold Cereals

Apple Jacks, Corn Flakes, Rice Krispies, Corn Pops, Corn Chex, Honey Comb, Honey Snacks, and stuffed rice. Select cereal options that are free from added dried fruits, nuts, raisins, or granola. (Serve with non-dairy liquid creamer instead of milk.

Miscellaneous

Butter, margarine, olive oil, canola oil, cream cheese, sour cream, and Italian dressing Non-dairy whipped topping. Jelly, jam Sugar alternatives Catchup, mayo mustard, salad dressing, and sherbert sorbet.

Sweets

- Apple Spread
- A variety of cakes like sponge, lemon, and spice
- Seasonal candy corn
- Flavorful chewing gum
- Sweet cinnamon treats
- An assortment of cookies, including sugar, gingersnap, and lemon cream
- Whimsical cotton candy
- Doughnuts, minus the nuts and chocolate
- Refreshing fruit ice
- Jiggly gelatin
- Colorful gumdrops
- Crunchy hard candies
- Natural honey and spreads
- Fruity jelly beans
- Rich maple syrup
- Citrusy marmalade

- Soft marshmallows
- Classic peppermints
- Pies filled with fruits like apple and cherry
- Chilled fruit popsicles
- Crunchy Rice Krispie treats
- Chewy red licorice
- Sweet sorbet
- Crisp vanilla wafers
- Delightful vanilla cupcakes

5 Tips for Making a Diabetic Kidney Disease Diet Work for You

1. Choose the Right Stuff to Eat
- *Veggies:* Go for lots of fresh vegetables like peppers, broccoli, and carrots. They're good for your kidneys and blood sugar.
- *Fruits:* Snack on fruits like apples and watermelon. Berries are awesome because they don't have much sugar.
- *Whole Grains:* Foods like whole grain bread and brown rice are great because they don't mess with your blood sugar too much.
- *Proteins:* Eat fresh proteins like chicken and fish. Stay away from processed stuff like sausages because they have too much salt and other things that aren't good for your kidneys.

- **Fats:** Not all fats are bad. Unsaturated fats, like those in nuts and fish, are good for you.

2. Watch Out for the Bad Stuff
- Avoid too much salt as it can raise your blood pressure and hurt your kidneys.
- Be careful with potassium and phosphorus; your body struggles to balance these if you have kidney issues.
- Too many sweets are a no-go because they can mess up your diabetes control.

3. Don't Skip Meals: Missing meals can make your blood sugar levels go crazy. Eat three good meals and some snacks every day to keep things steady.

4. Make Food Fun: Your diet doesn't have to be boring. Spice up your meals with herbs, spices, and some lemon or lime to add flavor without the salt.

5. Plan Yummy Meals: You can still enjoy eating. Use cookbooks with recipes that are good for your health. Look for healthier versions of your favorite dishes that fit your diabetes and kidney care plan.

©Nancy K. Doctor

CHAPTER 2

APPETIZERS AND BREAKFAST IDEAS

Spicy Tofu Scrambler

Serves: 2 (1 serving = ½ cup) | **Prep time: 10 minutes** | *Total time: 30 minutes*

<u>Ingredients:</u>
- 1 teaspoon olive oil
- ¼ cup red bell pepper, chopped
- ¼ cup green bell pepper, chopped
- one cup of dense tofu with a calcium content below 10%
- 1 teaspoon onion powder
- ¼ teaspoon garlic powder
- 1 clove garlic, minced
- ⅛ teaspoon turmeric

<u>Directions:</u>
1. In a saucepan of medium dimensions with a nonstick surface, proceed to cook the garlic along with the red and green bell peppers using olive oil.
2. Rinse and drain tofu and crumble it into the skillet. Add the remaining ingredients.

3. Go ahead and give everything a gentle mix while keeping the flame somewhere between low and medium. You're aiming to see the tofu get just a touch of golden brown color, which should take around 20 minutes. As it cooks, you'll notice the water in the mix will start to disappear.

TIP:
Make sure to peek at the nutrition facts and pick tofu varieties that have less than a 10% calcium content.

Renal-Friendly Garden Veggie Frittata

Cooking Time: 15 minutes (Prep: 5 mins, Cook: 10 mins) | Serving Size: 2 servings
Ingredients:
- 4 medium eggs
- 1 tablespoon of freshly chopped parsley, or 1 teaspoon of the dried variety
- ½ tsp dried oregano
- ¼ tsp garlic salt
- A dash of black pepper
- 1 tbsp water
- 2 tsp coconut oil
- 2 stalks green onion, chopped

- ½ cup raw broccoli (or asparagus, green beans)
- ½ cup diced celery

Directions:
1. Whisk eggs, parsley, oregano, garlic salt, pepper, and water in a bowl.
2. Sauté green onions, broccoli, and celery in melted coconut oil over medium heat until tender.
3. Add egg mixture to the pan, cover, and cook until eggs are set.

Note/Tips:
- Experiment with various veggies like mushrooms, cauliflower, or bell peppers.
- Substitute garlic salt with a mix of sea salt and garlic powder.
- Store it in a sealed container in the fridge for a duration of three to four days.

Cranberry Almond Bulgur Cereal

Prep Time: 10 minutes | Cooking Time: 6 minutes | Serving Size: ½ cup per serving

Ingredients:
- 1 cup Bulgur wheat
- 1 cup Cranergy drink (or any cranberry energy drink)
- 1 tablespoon sugar
- 1 tablespoon cinnamon

- ½ cup Craisins (dried cranberries)
- ¼ cup almonds, chopped

Instructions:

1. In a microwave-safe bowl, combine the bulgur wheat, Cranergy drink, sugar, and cinnamon. Stir the ingredients together until everything is evenly mixed.
2. Place a lid or plate that is suitable for microwave use atop the bowl. Microwave on high for 5 minutes, or until all the liquid has been absorbed by the bulgur. Exercise caution when taking the bowl out of the microwave as it will be hot.
3. Once cooked, remove the cover and fluff the bulgur with a fork. Stir in the Craisins, distributing them evenly throughout the cereal.
4. To serve, sprinkle the chopped almonds over the top of the cereal for added texture and a nutty flavor.
5. Serve the cereal warm, providing a hearty and nutritious start to your day. If desired, you can add a splash of milk or a dollop of yogurt for extra creaminess.

©Nancy K. Doctor

Charred Red Bell Pepper Chickpea Spread

Number of Servings: Serves 16
Ingredients:
- Two cups of rinsed and drained canned chickpeas
- 1 cup of roasted red bell pepper slices, seeded
- 2 tablespoons of white sesame seeds
- 1 tablespoon of lemon juice
- 1 tablespoon of olive oil
- 1¼ teaspoons of cumin
- 1 teaspoon of onion powder
- 1 teaspoon of garlic powder
- 1 teaspoon of kosher salt
- ¼ teaspoon of cayenne pepper

Directions:
In a food processor, blend all the ingredients until the mixture achieves a smooth consistency.

Tangy Asparagus Spears

Number of Servings: Serves 6
Ingredients:
- 1 pound of fresh asparagus, ends trimmed (approximately 3 cups)
- ¼ cup of pearl onions

- ¼ cup of white wine vinegar
- ¼ cup of cider vinegar
- 1 sprig of fresh dill (or 2 teaspoons dried)
- 1 cup of water
- 2 whole cloves
- 3 whole garlic cloves
- 8 whole black peppercorns
- ¼ teaspoon of red pepper flakes
- 6 whole coriander seeds

Directions:

1. Prepare the asparagus by trimming off the tough, woody ends and cutting the spears to fit your jars.
2. Clean the asparagus spears thoroughly in a strainer, rinse well, and let them drain. Also, trim the pearl onions as needed.
3. In air-tight containers, combine the trimmed asparagus, pearl onions, white wine vinegar, cider vinegar, fresh dill, water, whole cloves, garlic cloves, black peppercorns, red pepper flakes, and coriander seeds.
4. Ensure the jars are sealed tightly and refrigerated. The pickled asparagus will be ready to enjoy for up to 4 weeks.

Creamy Peanut Butter Chickpea Dip

Number of Servings: 16 servings
Ingredients:
- 2 cups of chickpeas (garbanzo beans)
- 1 cup of water
- ½ cup of powdered peanut butter
- ¼ cup of natural peanut butter
- 2 tablespoons of brown sugar
- 1 teaspoon of vanilla extract

Preparation Instructions:
1. Combine the chickpeas, water, powdered peanut butter, natural peanut butter, brown sugar, and vanilla extract in a food processor.
2. Process the mixture until it reaches a smooth texture.
3. Transfer the dip to a container and refrigerate. It can be stored and enjoyed for up to one week.

Tip:
This versatile dip is perfect for spreading on sandwiches or as a delightful dip for fruits and vegetables.

Classic Chickpea Spread

Number of Servings: 14 servings.
Ingredients:
- 2 cans (each 16 ounces) of low-sodium chickpeas, keep ¼ cup of the liquid and rinse and drain the rest
- 1 tablespoon of extra-virgin olive oil
- ¼ cup of lemon juice
- 2 cloves of garlic, minced
- ¼ teaspoon of cracked black pepper
- ¼ teaspoon of paprika
- 3 tablespoons of tahini (sesame paste)
- 2 tablespoons of chopped Italian flat-leaf parsley

Preparation Instructions:
- In a blender or food processor, start by pureeing the chickpeas until smooth.
- Gradually add in the olive oil, lemon juice, minced garlic, black pepper, paprika, tahini, and parsley, blending well after each addition.
- To achieve the desired consistency of a thick spread, incorporate the reserved chickpea liquid, adding 1 tablespoon at a time.
- The hummus can be served immediately or stored in the refrigerator, covered until it's time to enjoy.

©Nancy K. Doctor

Grilled Veggie Avocado Dip

Prep: 10 mins | Cook Time: 8 mins | Serving Size: 8 servings

Ingredients:
- 2 tbsp Canola oil (divided)
- 1 small Zucchini (cut lengthwise into 3 strips)
- 1 medium Red bell pepper (halved, seeds removed)
- 1 Avocado (halved, peeled)
- ½ small Red onion (sliced)
- Juice of 1 whole lime
- ¼ cup Cilantro (minced)
- 8 cups Salted white corn tortilla chips

Directions:
1. Brush the grill with canola oil and preheat to medium-high.
2. Lightly oil vegetables with 1 tbsp canola oil.
3. Grill zucchini, bell pepper, avocado, and onion for 3-4 minutes per side.
4. Dice grilled zucchini, pepper, and onion; place in a bowl.
5. Mash in avocado.
6. Stir in the remaining oil, lime juice, and cilantro. Chill before serving.

Tips:
Avocados are rich in monounsaturated fatty acids, beneficial for heart health.

Spinach and Mushroom Egg Cups

Cooking Time: Approx. 20-25 mins | Serving Size: Varies (based on the number of muffin cups)

Ingredients:
- Eggs (number based on muffin cups used)
- Fresh spinach, chopped
- Mushrooms, sliced
- Salt and pepper to taste
- Optional: low-sodium cheese, herbs for flavor

Directions:
1. Preheat the oven to 350°F (175°C). Grease the muffin tin cups lightly.
2. Place a few spinach leaves and mushroom slices in each muffin cup.
3. Crack an egg into each cup. Season with salt and pepper.
4. Optionally, sprinkle a small amount of low-sodium cheese or herbs for added flavor.
5. Bake in the preheated oven for 15-20 minutes, or until the eggs are set to your liking.

Dietician's Tips:
- Adjust the baking time depending on how you prefer your eggs.

- Ensure to use fresh ingredients for the best taste and nutritional value.

Oven-Baked Yogurt and Lemon Chicken Nuggets

Prep Time: 40 mins | Marinating Time: 4 hours | Cooking Time: 20 mins | Serving Size: 5 nuggets per serving

Ingredients:

- 1.5 pounds of chicken breast, sliced into nuggets measuring 1.5 by 1 inches
- 1 6-ounce container of low-sodium, low-fat Greek yogurt
- ½ cup lemon juice
- 1 cup all-purpose white flour
- 1 egg, whisked
- A cup of crushed wheat corn flakes or unsalted corn chips
- ¼ teaspoon dried dill
- ¼ teaspoon dried celery seed
- ¼ teaspoon salt-free garlic powder
- ¼ teaspoon dried lemon peel
- ¼ teaspoon freshly ground black pepper
- Olive oil spray

Instructions:

1. In a plastic container, thoroughly mix the chicken nuggets with the Greek yogurt and

lemon juice. Make certain that the marinade thoroughly covers every segment. Cover the container and refrigerate overnight, or for a minimum of four hours, to marinate.

2. Before beginning the cooking process, ensure your oven is preheated to 400 degrees Fahrenheit (200°C). It is important to let the chicken sit until it is at room temperature before applying the coating.
3. Prepare your breading station with three separate bowls: the first with flour, the second with the whisked egg, and the third with crushed cornflakes mixed with the spices (dill, celery seed, garlic powder, lemon peel, and black pepper).
4. Place an oven-safe cooling rack over a baking sheet, or line the baking sheet with parchment paper if you don't have a cooling rack.
5. Bread each chicken nugget by first coating it in flour, then dipping it in the egg, and finally rolling it in the spiced cornflake mixture. Arrange the breaded nuggets on the cooling rack or baking sheet.
6. Lightly spray the breaded nuggets with olive oil to encourage browning and crispiness. Bake in the preheated oven for 15 to 20 minutes, or until the nuggets are golden brown and crispy.

7. Serve the chicken nuggets warm, ideally with a side of fresh vegetables or a dipping sauce of your choice.

Peanut Butter Infused Oatmeal Bliss

Prep Time: 10 minutes | Cooking Time: 10 minutes | Serving size: ⅔ Cup Per Serving

Ingredients:
- 1⅓ cups uncooked oatmeal
- 4 tablespoons peanut butter
- ¼ cup honey

Preparation:
1. Prepare oatmeal in water according to the package instructions, excluding the salt.
2. Separate the prepared oatmeal evenly among four dishes, incorporating a tablespoon of peanut butter and a tablespoon of honey into every serving.

©Nancy K. Doctor

BEVERAGE AND SMOOTHIES

Refreshing Lime and Mint Tea

Number of Servings: Serves 1 person
Ingredients:
- 1 cup of freshly brewed unsweetened tea, cooled
- 2 tablespoons of lime juice concentrate
- 2 tablespoons of fresh mint leaves, plus an additional sprig for garnish
- 5 to 6 ice cubes
- Sugar substitute to taste

Preparation Instructions:
1. In a blender, combine the cooled tea, lime juice concentrate, fresh mint leaves, and ice cubes.
2. Blend the mixture until it becomes smooth and frothy.
3. Taste the blend and add a sugar substitute according to your preference for sweetness.
4. Pour the tea into a tall, chilled glass.
5. Top it off with a mint leaf to add a bit of class.

Dietitian's Tip:
For those who prefer brewed tea, you can prepare it by heating water until it simmers, then removing it from the heat and adding the tea. Use 1 teaspoon of tea per 1 cup of water. This recipe can be made with either cooled brewed tea or instant tea, depending on your preference.

Refreshing Lime Mockarita

Number of Servings: Serves 2 people.
Ingredients:
For the **Simple Syrup:**
- ½ cup of sugar
- ½ cup of water

For the **Margaritas:**
- 2 cups of ice
- ½ cup of fresh lime juice
- 3 tablespoons of the prepared simple syrup
- Fresh fruit slices for garnish (optional)

Preparation Instructions:
1. To whip up a batch of sweet syrup, just mix some sugar and water in a little pot. Heat the mixture, stirring constantly, until the sugar has completely dissolved. Remove from heat and allow it to chill in the refrigerator.
2. In a blender, combine the ice, fresh lime juice, and 3 tablespoons of the chilled

simple syrup. Blend until the mixture is smooth.

3. Pour the blended mockarita into your favorite chilled glasses. If desired, garnish the rim of each glass with a slice of fresh fruit for an extra touch of elegance.

Dietitian's Tip:

This recipe produces more simple *syrup than required.* Store the excess in the refrigerator for up to several days to use in other beverages or recipes.

Strawberry Lime Bliss

Number of Servings: Serves 6
Ingredients:
- 4 cups of sliced strawberries
- ¼ cup of lime juice
- ¼ cup of sugar (consider a sugar substitute for a lower-calorie option)
- 2 cups of water
- 2 cups of ice

Preparation Instructions:
1. Combine the sliced strawberries, lime juice, sugar (or sugar substitute), water, and ice in a blender.
2. Process the mixture until it reaches a smooth texture.

3. Serve the Strawberry Lime Bliss immediately, ensuring its refreshing taste is enjoyed at its best.

Dietitian's Tip:
This nonalcoholic cocktail is an excellent choice for both starting and ending your meal on a refreshing note. For those monitoring their sugar intake, substituting sugar with a low-calorie sweetener can make this drink suitable for a diabetic diet without compromising on the taste.

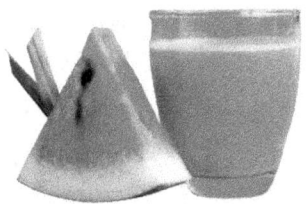

©Nancy K. Doctor

PASTRY/DESSERT

Savory Chicken Zucchini Pie

Prep Time: 40 minutes, Cooking Time: 1 hour
Ingredients:
- 9-inch pie crust, ready to bake
- 6 oz. ground chicken
- 1½ (6 oz.) zucchinis, chopped
- 2 teaspoons of sage, ground
- ½ teaspoon of onion powder
- 5 large eggs
- 1 cup of rice milk
- 1 tablespoon of poultry seasoning
- 3 slices of Swiss cheese

Instructions:
1. Preheat your oven to 350°F (175°C). Fit the pie crust into a pie plate, pressing it into the corners and trimming any excess dough from the edges.
2. In a medium skillet over medium heat, cook the ground chicken with the diced zucchini, ground sage, and onion powder until the chicken is fully cooked. Take it off the stove and let it chill out until it's as cool as the room you're in.

3. In a separate bowl, whisk together the eggs, rice milk, and poultry seasoning until well combined.
4. Spread the cooled chicken and zucchini mixture evenly over the bottom of the pie crust. Gently pour the egg mixture over the chicken and zucchini.
5. Cut the Swiss cheese slices in half and arrange them on top of the egg mixture, ensuring even coverage.
6. Bake in the preheated oven on the lowest rack for 50 to 60 minutes, or until the edges of the crust are golden brown and the center of the quiche is set and no longer runny.
7. After baking, allow the quiche to cool for 10 minutes on a wire rack before slicing into 8 portions and serving.

Nutritious Whole-Grain Soda Bread

Number of Servings: Serves 16
Ingredients:
- 2 cups of whole-wheat flour
- 1 teaspoon of baking powder
- ¼ cup of flaxseed meal (ground flaxseed)
- ½ teaspoon of baking soda
- ¼ cup of millet meal (ground millet)

- 1 teaspoon of crushed caraway seed
- 2 tablespoons of wheat gluten
- ¼ teaspoon of kosher salt
- 1¼ cups of low-fat buttermilk or skim milk (for a plant-based option, use a suitable milk substitute)
- 2 egg whites (for a plant-based option, use an appropriate egg substitute)

Preparation Instructions:

1. Preheat your oven to 350°F (175°C).
2. In a large mixing bowl, sift together the whole-wheat flour, baking powder, flaxseed meal, baking soda, millet meal, crushed caraway seed, wheat gluten, and kosher salt.
3. In a separate bowl, whisk together the low-fat buttermilk (or milk substitute) and egg whites (or egg substitute) until well combined.
4. Gradually add the wet ingredients to the dry ingredients, stirring until the mixture is evenly moistened.
5. Lightly grease the bottom of a 5-by-8-inch loaf pan and transfer the dough into the pan. With a sharp knife, make a longitudinal slash about ¼ inch deep on the top of the dough.
6. Place it in the oven and let it cook for a good 50 to 60 minutes. You'll know it's done when you poke the middle of the bread with

a skewer and it pulls out without any gooey bits sticking to it.

Dietitian's Tip:
This recipe can be made plant-based by substituting the milk and egg with suitable alternatives.

Mixed-Grain Raspberry Muffins

Number of Servings: Makes 12 muffins.
Ingredients:
- ½ cup of rolled oats
- 1 cup of 1 percent low-fat milk or plain soy milk (for a plant-based option)
- ¾ cup of all-purpose flour
- ½ cup of cornmeal (coarse-ground preferred)
- ¼ cup of wheat bran
- 1 tablespoon of baking powder
- ¼ teaspoon of salt
- ½ cup of honey (or maple syrup for a plant-based option)
- 3½ tablespoons of canola oil
- 2 teaspoons of grated lime zest
- 1 egg, lightly beaten (or an egg substitute for a plant-based option)
- ⅔ cup of raspberries

Preparation Instructions:

1. Preheat the oven to 400°F (200°C). Get your 12-cup muffin tin ready by popping in some paper or foil cups.
2. In a large microwave-safe bowl, mix the oats and milk. Heat the oats in the microwave at full power until they achieve a creamy consistency and soft texture, which should take approximately 3 minutes. Set aside to cool slightly.
3. In a separate large bowl, whisk together the flour, cornmeal, wheat bran, baking powder, and salt.
4. Stir in the honey (or maple syrup), canola oil, lime zest, the oat-milk mixture, and the beaten egg (or egg substitute) into the dry ingredients until just moistened but still slightly lumpy. Carefully fold in the raspberries.
5. Spoon the batter into the prepared muffin cups, filling each about ⅔ full.
6. Bake for 16 to 18 minutes, or until the tops are golden brown and a toothpick inserted into the center of a muffin comes out clean.
7. Cool the muffins on a wire rack before serving or storing.

Dietitian's Tip:

These muffins can be stored in the freezer in a lock-top plastic bag if you have extras. This makes them a convenient and quick breakfast or snack option for busy days.

Warmly Spiced Carrot and Raisin Loaf

Number of Servings: Serves 18
Ingredients:
- 1½ cups of whole-wheat pastry flour
- ¼ cup of flaxseed flour
- ½ teaspoon of baking soda
- 1½ teaspoons of baking powder
- ½ teaspoon of salt
- 1 tablespoon of cinnamon
- ½ teaspoon of nutmeg
- ¼ teaspoon of cloves
- ¼ teaspoon of ground cayenne pepper
- 2 eggs (or an egg substitute for a plant-based option)
- ½ cup of brown sugar
- ¼ cup of honey (or maple syrup for a plant-based option)
- ½ cup of unsweetened applesauce
- ¼ cup of olive oil
- ¾ teaspoon of almond extract
- 1 tablespoon of grated lemon zest
- 2 cups of shredded carrots (about 4 medium carrots)

- ⅔ cup of raisins

Preparation Instructions:
1. Preheat your oven to 375°F (190°C). Lightly grease a 9-by-5-inch loaf pan.
2. In a large bowl, sift together the whole-wheat pastry flour, flaxseed flour, baking soda, baking powder, salt, cinnamon, nutmeg, cloves, and cayenne pepper. Blend the dry components thoroughly until they are uniformly mixed.
3. In a separate bowl, whisk together the eggs (or egg substitute), brown sugar, honey (or maple syrup), applesauce, olive oil, and almond extract. Stir in the lemon zest, shredded carrots, and raisins.
4. Gradually mix the wet ingredients into the dry ingredients, stirring just until combined. Be careful not to overmix.
5. Pour the batter into the prepared loaf pan. Place the loaf in the oven and let it cook for a duration of 45 to 60 minutes. The bread is done when a toothpick, after being inserted into the middle of the loaf, emerges without any batter attached.
6. Give the bread time to settle and cool down slightly in the pan before moving it onto a wire rack, where it should be left to cool entirely.

Dietitian's Tip:
Flaxseed flour and a blend of spices, including a hint of cayenne pepper, give this tea bread its rich flavor and moist texture. For a plant-based version, substitute the honey with maple syrup and use an appropriate egg substitute.

Savory Southwestern Cornmeal Muffins

Number of Servings: Makes 12 muffins
Ingredients:
- 1 cup of all-purpose flour
- ¼ cup of sugar
- 2 teaspoons of baking powder
- 1 cup of fat-free milk (or a plant-based milk substitute)
- 4 tablespoons (¼ cup) of vegetable oil
- ½ cup of egg substitute (or a plant-based egg alternative)
- 1¼ cups of stone-ground cornmeal
- 1 cup of fresh or cream-style corn
- ½ green bell pepper, finely chopped

Preparation Instructions:
1. Preheat your oven to 400°F (200°C). Get your 12-cup muffin tin ready by popping in some paper or foil cups.

2. In a large mixing bowl, combine the flour, sugar, and baking powder, stirring well to ensure even distribution.
3. In a separate bowl, mix the milk, vegetable oil, egg substitute, cornmeal, corn, and chopped green bell pepper until well combined.
4. Combine the dry and wet elements, mixing only to the point where they're dampened and a bit clumpy. Then, portion out the batter into the muffin slots, filling each to about two-thirds of the way.
5. Bake for 20 minutes, or until the muffins are light brown and a toothpick inserted into the center of a muffin comes out clean.
6. Make sure you let those muffins chill out a bit before you dish them out.

Dietitian's Tip:

Stone-ground cornmeal is not only flavorful but also a good source of fiber, vitamin C, and potassium, making these muffins a nutritious choice. For a fully plant-based version, opt for milk and egg substitutes and consider using maple syrup instead of honey if sweetness adjustment is needed.

©Nancy K. Doctor

Wholesome Muesli Energy Bars

Number of Servings: Makes 24 bars

Ingredients:
- 2½ cups of old-fashioned rolled oats
- ½ cup of soy flour
- ½ cup of fat-free dry milk (or a vegan protein powder for a plant-based option)
- ½ cup of toasted wheat germ
- ½ cup of sliced almonds or chopped pecans toasted
- ½ cup of chopped dried apples
- ½ cup of raisins
- ½ teaspoon of salt
- 1 cup of dark honey (or maple syrup for a plant-based option)
- ½ cup of natural unsalted peanut butter
- 1 tablespoon of olive oil
- 2 teaspoons of vanilla extract

Preparation Instructions:
1. Preheat your oven to 325°F (163°C). Go ahead and give a 9x13-inch baking dish a quick spritz with some cooking spray.
2. In a large bowl, mix the rolled oats, soy flour, dry milk (or vegan protein powder), wheat germ, almonds (or pecans), dried apples, raisins, and salt until well combined.
3. In a small saucepan over medium-low heat, combine the honey (or maple syrup), peanut

butter, and olive oil. Stir until the mixture is well blended and warm, ensuring it does not boil. Take it off the stove and mix in the vanilla flavoring.
4. Quickly add the warm honey mixture to the dry ingredients, stirring until thoroughly combined. Your blend ought to have a tacky consistency without feeling overly damp.
5. Press the mixture evenly into the prepared baking pan, ensuring there are no air pockets.
6. Bake for about 25 minutes, or until the edges start to turn golden brown. Allow to cool in the pan on a wire rack for 10 minutes, then cut into 24 bars. Remove the bars from the pan while still warm and let them cool completely on the rack.
7. Keep your bars fresh by sealing them in containers that are airtight and popping them into the fridge.

Dietitian's Tip:

Cornmeal that's been ground with stones is packed with beneficial goodies like fiber, vitamin C, and a nice dose of potassium. For a fully plant-based version, opt for milk and egg substitutes and consider using maple syrup instead of honey if sweetness adjustment is needed.

©Nancy K. Doctor

Traditional Irish Whole-Wheat Bread

Number of Servings: Makes 24 slices
Ingredients:
- 2 cups of whole-wheat flour
- 1½ cups of all-purpose flour, plus extra for kneading and dusting
- ½ cup of wheat germ
- 2 teaspoons of baking soda
- ¼ teaspoon of salt
- 2 cups of low-fat buttermilk (or a plant-based milk substitute mixed with 1 tablespoon of lemon juice or vinegar to mimic buttermilk)
- 1 egg, lightly beaten (or a plant-based egg substitute)

Preparation Instructions:
1. Preheat your oven to 400°F (200°C) and prepare a nonstick baking sheet.
2. In a large mixing bowl, whisk together the whole-wheat flour, all-purpose flour, wheat germ, baking soda, and salt.
3. Stir in the buttermilk and egg until just moistened. The dough will be sticky.
4. Turn the dough onto a floured surface and gently knead it 8 to 10 times with floured

hands. Go ahead and gently form the dough into a relaxed, round shape.
5. Place the dough on the prepared baking sheet and form it into a 7-inch round. Lightly dust the top with flour and cut a large X, about ½ inch deep, across the top.
6. Bake for 25 to 30 minutes, or until the bread has split open at the X and sounds hollow when tapped underneath.
7. Transfer the bread to a wire rack to cool for at least 2 hours before slicing to allow the texture to develop fully.

Dietitian's Tip:
This traditional Irish bread is a staple that's rich in fiber and nutrients, thanks to the whole-wheat flour and wheat germ. For a plant-based version, substitute the buttermilk with a dairy-free alternative and use an egg substitute.

Berry Delight Whole-Grain Coffee Cake

Number of Servings: Serves 8
Ingredients:
- ½ cup of skim milk
- 1 tablespoon of vinegar
- 2 tablespoons of canola oil
- 1 teaspoon of vanilla extract

- 1 egg
- ⅓ cup of packed brown sugar
- 1 cup of whole-wheat pastry flour
- ½ teaspoon of baking soda
- ½ teaspoon of ground cinnamon
- ⅛ teaspoon of salt
- 1 cup of frozen mixed berries (blueberries, raspberries, blackberries), do not thaw
- ¼ cup of low-fat granola, slightly crushed

Preparation Instructions:

1. Preheat your oven to 350°F (175°C). Spray an 8-inch round cake pan with cooking spray and lightly coat it with flour.
2. In a large bowl, whisk together the milk, vinegar, canola oil, vanilla extract, egg, and brown sugar until smooth.
3. Stir in the whole-wheat pastry flour, baking soda, cinnamon, and salt just until the mixture is moistened.
4. Gently fold half of the berries into the batter, then spoon the batter into the prepared pan.
5. Sprinkle the remaining berries over the batter and top with the crushed granola.
6. Bake for 25 to 30 minutes, or until the cake is golden brown and springs back when touched in the center.
7. Let the cake sit in the pan atop a wire rack to chill for a good 10 minutes. Serve warm.

Dietitian's Tip:

Using whole-wheat pastry flour and fresh or frozen berries adds fiber and nutrients to this coffee cake, making it a healthier option. The combination of skim milk and canola oil keeps the fat content low while ensuring the cake remains moist and tender.

Rustic Apple-Cranberry Tart

Number of Servings: Serves 8
Ingredients:
For the Filling:
- ½ cup dried cranberries
- ¼ cup apple juice
- 1 teaspoon vanilla extract
- ¼ teaspoon ground cinnamon
- 2 tablespoons cornstarch
- 4 large tart apples (such as Granny Smith), cored, peeled, and sliced

For the Crust:
- 1¼ cups whole-wheat flour
- 2 teaspoons sugar
- 1½ tablespoons unsalted butter, melted
- 1½ tablespoons canola oil
- ¼ cup ice water

Preparation Instructions:
1. In a small microwave-safe bowl, combine cranberries and apple juice. Microwave on high for 1 minute, stir, and continue heating in 30-second intervals, stirring each time,

until the juice is very hot. Cover and set aside until near room temperature, about 1 hour. Stir in vanilla and cinnamon.
2. Preheat the oven to 375°F (190°C). In a large bowl, toss the apple slices with cornstarch until evenly coated. Go ahead and blend the cranberry concoction thoroughly.
3. In a large mixing bowl, whisk together the flour and sugar. Combine the melted butter and oil, then drizzle over the dry ingredients. The mixture will be crumbly. Gradually add ice water, mixing until the dough forms a rough mass.
4. On a floured piece of aluminum foil, roll the dough into a 13-inch diameter circle. Place the fruit filling in the center, leaving a 1- to 2-inch border. Flip the crust's borders over the top of the filling, making sure to keep the middle part uncovered.
5. Transfer the tart (with the bottom foil) onto a cookie sheet. Cover the exposed fruit with another piece of foil. Bake for about 30 minutes, remove the top foil, and bake until browned, about 10 more minutes.
6. Serve immediately, cut into 8 wedges.

Dietitian's Tip:
Tart-baking apples, such as Granny Smith or Northern Spy, hold their shape well in this rustic

tart. This dessert is sweet yet low in added sugar, making it a healthier option.

Spiced Carrot Raisin Loaf

Number of Servings: Serves 18
Ingredients:
- 1½ cups of whole-wheat pastry flour
- ¼ cup of flaxseed flour
- ½ teaspoon of baking soda
- 1½ teaspoons of baking powder
- ½ teaspoon of salt
- 1 tablespoon of cinnamon
- ½ teaspoon of nutmeg
- ¼ teaspoon of cloves
- ¼ teaspoon of ground cayenne pepper
- 2 eggs
- ½ cup of brown sugar
- ¼ cup of honey (or maple syrup for a plant-based option)
- ½ cup of unsweetened applesauce
- ¼ cup of olive oil
- ¾ teaspoon of almond extract
- 1 tablespoon of grated lemon zest
- 2 cups of shredded carrots (about 4 medium carrots)
- ⅔ cup of raisins

Preparation Instructions:

1. Preheat your oven to 375°F (190°C). Lightly grease a 9-by-5-inch loaf pan.
2. In a large bowl, sift together the whole-wheat pastry flour, flaxseed flour, baking soda, baking powder, salt, cinnamon, nutmeg, cloves, and cayenne pepper. Whisk to combine.
3. In a separate bowl, mix the eggs, brown sugar, honey (or maple syrup), applesauce, olive oil, and almond extract. Stir in the lemon zest, shredded carrots, and raisins.
4. Go ahead and mix the dry and wet ingredients, making sure to stir them only until they're nicely incorporated.
5. Pour the batter into the prepared loaf pan. Place it in the oven for about 45 to 60 minutes. You'll know it's ready when you poke the middle with a skewer and it comes out without any gooey bits.
6. Let it hang out in the pan for a bit to chill, then shift it over to a cooling grid to let it cool down all the way. Slice into ½-inch thick slices to serve.

Dietitian's Tip:
Flaxseed flour and a blend of spices, including a hint of cayenne pepper, give this tea bread its rich flavor and moist texture. For a fully plant-based version, opt for maple syrup instead of honey.

©Nancy K. Doctor

Wholesome Apple Pie

Number of Servings: Serves 8
Ingredients:
For the Pie Crust:
- 1 cup of dry rolled oats
- ¼ cup of whole-wheat pastry flour
- ¼ cup of ground almonds
- 2 tablespoons of brown sugar, packed
- 3 tablespoons of canola oil
- 1 tablespoon of water

For the Filling:
- 6 cups of tart apples that have been peeled and cut (approximately 4 sizable apples)
- ⅓ cup of frozen apple juice concentrate
- 2 tablespoons of quick-cooking tapioca
- 1 teaspoon of cinnamon

Preparation Instructions:

1. Prepare the Pie Crust: In a large mixing bowl, combine the dry ingredients (rolled oats, whole-wheat pastry flour, ground almonds, and brown sugar). In a separate bowl, whisk together the canola oil and water.

2. Add the oil and water mixture to the dry ingredients, mixing until the dough holds together. Add a bit more water if needed. Press the dough into a 9-inch pie plate and set aside.

3. Prepare the Filling: In another large bowl, combine the sliced apples, apple juice concentrate, tapioca, and cinnamon. Let the mixture stand for 15 minutes, then stir and spoon it into the prepared pie crust.
4. Bake the Pie: Preheat the oven to 425°F (220°C). Bake the pie for 15 minutes, then reduce the heat to 350°F (175°C) and continue baking for 40 minutes, or until the apples are tender.

Dietitian's Tip:
This pie crust, made with whole grains and almonds, offers a nutritious alternative to traditional pie crusts, being high in fiber. The filling, sweetened with apple juice concentrate, reduces the need for added sugars, making this pie a healthier option for those managing their sugar intake.

MAIN DISH/LUNCH

Seared Salmon with Braised Broccoli

Serving size: 4 servings | Prep time: 40 minutes | Total time: 40 minutes

Ingredients

- 1¼ pounds wild Alaskan salmon filet, skinned and cut into 4 portions
- 1 tablespoon of finely minced fresh rosemary, or one teaspoon of the dried variety
- 1 teaspoon salt, divided
- 2 heads broccoli, (1-1½ pounds), trimmed
- 1½ tablespoons extra-virgin olive oil, divided
- 1 small onion, diced
- 3 tablespoons raisins
- 2 tablespoons pine nuts
- ½ cup water

Directions:

1. Season the salmon using half of the allotted rosemary and a half teaspoon of salt, allowing it to marinate for a minimum of 20 minutes to a maximum of one hour before cooking.
2. Prepare the broccoli by separating it into florets, ensuring each has a 2-inch stalk attached. Use a vegetable peeler to strip away the fibrous exterior layer of the stalks. Cut the florets in half lengthwise.
3. Warm a tablespoon of oil in a spacious saucepan set over a medium flame. Incorporate the onion, periodically stirring, until it becomes semi-transparent, which should take about 3 to 4 minutes.

4. Add the raisins, pine nuts, and the rest of the rosemary, stirring them to ensure they are evenly covered in the oil. Cook, stirring, until the pine nuts are fragrant and beginning to brown 3 to 5 minutes.
5. Add the broccoli, season with the remaining ½ teaspoon salt, and toss to combine. Add water and bring to a boil.
6. Lower the temperature to sustain a soft simmer, stirring now and then, until the water is nearly gone, which should take about 8 to 10 minutes. Concurrently, warm the last half tablespoon of oil in a sizeable nonstick pan over a medium-high flame.
7. Place the salmon in the pan with the skin side facing up and sear until it achieves a golden hue, a process taking approximately 3 to 5 minutes.
8. Flip the salmon, withdraw the skillet from the stove, and let it rest until it reaches the desired doneness, which should be an additional 3 to 5 minutes.
9. To serve, divide the broccoli among 4 plates. Top with salmon and spoon raisins, pine nuts, and any liquid remaining in the pan over the salmon

Rosemary Infused Chicken Skewers

Cooking Time: 25 mins (+2 hours marinating time) Serving Size: 8 servings

Ingredients:
- 681 grams boneless, skinless chicken breast, trimmed and cut into 2-inch pieces
- 3 tablespoons extra virgin olive oil
- 2 tablespoons fresh rosemary
- A dash of black pepper
- 3 tablespoons lemon juice

Directions:
1. Clean skewers thoroughly with soap and water.
2. Mount the chicken segments onto metallic skewers.
3. Place skewers in a shallow, oven-safe baking dish.
4. Combine olive oil, lemon juice, rosemary, and pepper in a bowl.
5. Pour the marinade over the kebabs, using a brush to coat evenly.
6. Cover and refrigerate for 2 hours.
7. Preheat the broiler. Broil kebabs 3 inches from the heat for 10-15 minutes, until chicken is cooked through. Brush with

marinade in the first 5 minutes and turn frequently.
8. Serve hot and enjoy!

Note/Tips:
- *In case olive oil isn't on hand, you can go for avocado oil instead – it's an awesome substitute.*
- *Ensure chicken is thoroughly cooked to a safe internal temperature.*

Oven-Baked Salmon with Asparagus on Whole-Grain Bun

Prep Time: 45 minutes | Servings: 3 oz per serving

Ingredients:
- 16 oz. of fresh salmon filet
- 1 tablespoon of lemon juice
- 1 tablespoon of butter
- 12 oz. of fresh asparagus spears, tough ends trimmed and cleaned
- 1 tablespoon of olive oil
- 4 whole-grain or cracked wheat hamburger buns, lightly toasted

Instructions:
1. Heat your oven to 400°F (200°C) in preparation for roasting.
2. Place the asparagus spears on a baking sheet and drizzle them lightly with olive oil. Make

sure they are evenly spread out for consistent cooking.
3. Roast the asparagus in the preheated oven for about 10 minutes, or until they become tender and show signs of browning. Upon completion, take it out of the oven and let it stand for a brief period to cool down a bit.
4. Meanwhile, season the salmon filet with lemon juice and a touch of butter for added flavor.

Couscous Stuffed Peppers

Prep Time: 20 minutes | Cook Time: 1hr | Servings: 8 pepper halves

Ingredients:
- 1 cup low-sodium chicken broth
- 2 tsp ground cumin
- ¾ cup couscous
- 1 15oz can low sodium garbanzo beans rinsed
- ¼ cup dried cranberries
- 1 cup spinach packed
- ½ cup feta crumbled
- ¼ cup olive oil
- ½ tsp black pepper
- 4 bell peppers of any preferred hue, slice them in half along their length and remove the seeds

- 1 cup fresh basil leaves
- ½ cup sour cream
- 1 tablespoon water
- 1 clove garlic
- 2 teaspoons lemon juice
- ¼ teaspoon sugar
- ¼ teaspoon salt
- ¼ teaspoon black pepper

Instructions:
1. Preheat the oven to 400°F.
2. Make filling. Begin by heating the broth and cumin in a saucepan until it reaches a rolling boil. Take the pan off the heat and mix in the couscous. Seal the pan with a lid and leave it to stand for 5-6 minutes, or until the couscous has absorbed all the liquid. Using a fork, gently separate the grains of the couscous.
3. Next, incorporate the beans, dried cranberries, fresh spinach, crumbled feta cheese, a drizzle of olive oil, and a pinch of pepper into the couscous, stirring until everything is evenly distributed.
4. Proceed to fill the peppers with the prepared couscous mixture.
5. Pour water into a baking dish until it is half full, and nestle the stuffed peppers into the water. Transfer the dish to the oven and bake for 55-60 minutes, or until the filling turns a

golden brown hue and the peppers are tender.

6. While the peppers are baking, prepare the accompanying sauce. In a blender, combine fresh basil, sour cream, water, garlic, lemon juice, a dash of sugar, salt, and ground black pepper. Blend until smooth and creamy. Drizzle sauce over peppers before serving.

Low Sodium Stir Fry

Prep Time: 45 minutes | Cook Time: 20 minutes | Servings: 6 cup

Ingredients:
- ¾ pound pork tenderloin thinly sliced
- ½ head broccoli cut into florets
- 1 red bell pepper sliced
- 1 8 oz can water chestnuts drained
- 2 Tbsp low sodium soy sauce
- 2 teaspoons vegetable oil
- 2 cloves garlic minced
- 2 inches fresh ginger peeled and grated
- 2 green onions chopped
- 1 cup low-sodium chicken broth
- 2 tablespoons cornstarch
- 2 tablespoons low-sodium soy sauce
- 2 tablespoons hoisin sauce
- 2 tablespoons dry sherry
- 3 cups brown rice cooked

Instructions:

1. Blend two tablespoons of reduced-sodium soy sauce with vegetable oil, minced garlic, grated ginger, and chopped scallions. Add pork to marinade. Let sit for 30 minutes.
2. Meanwhile, blanch broccoli. Make sauce by whisking together broth, cornstarch, additional 2 tablespoons of low-sodium soy sauce, hoisin sauce, and sherry. Set aside.
3. Drain marinade from pork. Discard the marinade.
4. Warm up a teaspoon of veggie oil in your pan. Toss in the pork and give it a quick sear until it's no longer pink, which should take around a minute. Once done, move it over to a dish.
5. Now, grab another teaspoon of that oil and heat it in the skillet. Throw in your broccoli, peppers, and water chestnuts. Give them a good stir-fry until they've got a nice bite to them. Next, bring the pork back into the mix along with your sauce. Let everything simmer together until that sauce gets nice and thick, which should be about 3 minutes or so.
6. Serve 1 cup stir fry over ½ cup rice. Garnish with additional green onion if desired.

©Nancy K. Doctor

Nutritious Blueberry Whole-Wheat Pancakes

Number of Servings: Serves 6
Ingredients:
- 1⅓ cups of white whole-wheat flour
- 2 teaspoons of baking powder
- 1 tablespoon of sugar
- ½ teaspoon of cinnamon
- 1⅓ cups of skim milk (or a plant-based milk substitute for a vegan option)
- 1 egg, lightly beaten (or a plant-based egg substitute)
- 1 tablespoon of canola oil
- 1 cup of fresh or frozen blueberries

Preparation Instructions:
1. In a large mixing bowl, combine the flour, baking powder, sugar, and cinnamon.
2. In a separate bowl, whisk together the milk, egg (or egg substitute), and canola oil.
3. Add the liquid ingredients to the dry ingredients, stirring just until the flour is moistened. Be careful not to overmix.
4. Gently fold in the blueberries.
5. Warm up a griddle or frying pan on medium-high, and give it a quick spritz with some non-stick spray.

6. Then, ladle out roughly ¼ cup of the pancake mixture onto the sizzling surface for each flapjack. Cook until the edges are dry and bubbles form on the surface, then flip and cook until browned on the other side.

Dietitian's Tip:
White whole-wheat flour offers a smoother texture than regular whole-wheat flour, making it a great choice for pancakes. It provides the nutritional benefits of whole grains without compromising on texture or taste. For a plant-based version, substitute the milk and egg with your preferred alternatives.

Ultimate Vegetable Stir-Fry

Number of Servings: Serves 4
Ingredients:
- 1 teaspoon of sesame oil
- 1 medium onion, sliced
- 1 red bell pepper, chopped
- 1 green bell pepper, chopped
- 2 teaspoons of chopped fresh ginger
- 1 container (8 ounces) of button mushrooms, sliced
- 1 green onion, chopped
- 2 teaspoons of chopped fresh garlic
- 1 crown of broccoli, chopped into florets

- One big carrot peeled and cut into semi-circular shapes
- one tablespoon of sweet mirin, a traditional Japanese rice wine
- 1 tablespoon of reduced-sodium soy sauce
- 2 tablespoons of chopped cashews

Preparation Instructions:

1. Warm a nonstick frying pan on medium heat, then pour in the sesame oil. Once hot, add the onion, red and green bell peppers, and ginger. Sauté for 2 to 3 minutes.
2. Add the mushrooms, green onion, and garlic to the pan. Cook until the vegetables are tender.
3. Add the broccoli and carrots to the pan. Cover with a lid for 2 to 3 minutes to steam the vegetables until tender.
4. Stir in the mirin and soy sauce, mixing well to combine all the ingredients.
5. Sprinkle the chopped cashews over the stir-fry just before serving.

Dietitian's Tip:

This stir-fry is an excellent way to use up leftover vegetables in your refrigerator. It's a versatile dish that can be adapted to include your favorite vegetables or whatever you have on hand. Adding a protein source like tofu, chicken, or shrimp can turn it into a complete meal.

©Nancy K. Doctor

Sweet Potato Waffles with Homemade Blueberry Syrup

Number of Servings: Serves 6
Ingredients:
For the Blueberry Syrup:
- 1½ cups fresh or frozen blueberries
- 2 tablespoons water (if using fresh berries)
- 1 tablespoon fresh lemon juice
- 1 teaspoon grated lemon zest
- 1 tablespoon honey (or maple syrup for a plant-based option)
- 1 tablespoon light molasses
- A pinch of ground cloves

For the Waffles:
- ⅓ cup peeled and diced sweet potato (about ⅓ of a large sweet potato) or ¼ cup canned pumpkin puree
- ¾ cup all-purpose flour
- ¼ cup whole-wheat flour
- ¼ cup cornmeal, preferably stone-ground
- 1 tablespoon baking powder
- ½ teaspoon salt
- ⅛ teaspoon ground cinnamon
- ⅛ teaspoon ground ginger
- 1 cup plain soy milk (or any plant-based milk)
- 2 tablespoons light molasses

- 2 tablespoons olive oil
- 1 egg white (or a plant-based egg substitute)

Preparation Instructions:

1. Merge blueberries, optional water, freshly squeezed lemon juice, grated lemon zest, your choice of honey or maple syrup, dark molasses, and whole cloves in a cooking pot. Bring to a boil over medium-high heat, then reduce to low and simmer until berries burst and the sauce thickens about 5 minutes. Set aside and keep warm.
2. Boil diced sweet potato until tender, about 10 minutes. Drain and puree in a food processor or mash until smooth. Set aside to cool (Omit this phase if utilizing canned pumpkin puree).
3. In a bowl, sift together flour, cornmeal, baking powder, salt, cinnamon, and ginger. In another bowl, whisk together soy milk, mashed sweet potato (or pumpkin puree), olive oil, and molasses. Combine wet and dry ingredients.
4. Beat the egg white until stiff peaks form. Fold ⅓ of the egg white into the batter to lighten it, then gently fold in the remaining egg white.
5. Heat a waffle iron and cook the waffles according to the manufacturer's instructions.

6. Hold your waffles cozy in the oven until it's time to dish them out. Serve with the warm blueberry syrup.

Dietitian's Tip:
Sweet potatoes add a nutritional boost to these waffles, providing fiber, vitamins, and minerals. Blueberry syrup is a healthier alternative to traditional syrups, offering antioxidants and less added sugar.

Scalloped Corn-Stuffed Bell Peppers

Number of Servings: Serves 4
***Ingredients*:**
- 4 red or green bell peppers
- 1 tablespoon olive oil
- ½ onion, chopped (about ¼ cup)
- 1 green bell pepper, chopped
- 2½ cups fresh corn kernels (cut from about 4 large ears of corn)
- ⅛ teaspoon chili powder
- 2 tablespoons chopped fresh cilantro or parsley
- 3 egg whites
- ½ cup skim milk (or a plant-based milk substitute)
- ½ cup water

Preparation Instructions:
1. Preheat the oven to 350°F (175°C). Spritz a baking dish with a bit of non-stick spray. Slice off the tops of the bell peppers, scoop out the seeds, and nestle the peppers into the dish you just prepped.
2. Warm up some olive oil in a skillet over a medium flame. Toss in the diced onion, chopped green pepper, and sweet corn kernels. Give them a good stir-fry until they're nice and soft, which should take about 5 minutes.
3. Next, mix in a dash of chili powder and a handful of fresh cilantro or parsley, if you prefer. Turn down the heat so it's just a gentle simmer.
4. Grab a small bowl and beat the egg whites with some milk until well combined. Pour this egg white combo into the skillet with the veggies, turn the heat up a notch, and keep stirring. You're aiming for the egg whites to start firming up, but you want them still a tad runny, roughly 5 minutes of cooking.
5. Now, take your skillet and fill each pepper with an even share of the corn and egg white blend. Pour a little water into the base of your baking dish; this will help keep the peppers moist while they bake.

6. And there you have it, your stuffed peppers are ready to go into the oven!
7. Cover the peppers loosely with aluminum foil and bake until the peppers are tender about 15 minutes.
8. Serve the stuffed peppers on individual plates.

Dietitian's Tip:
For extra flavor, consider using roasted red bell peppers as the shells. Roasting enhances the sweetness of the peppers and adds a smoky depth to the dish. This recipe is also easily adaptable to be plant-based by using milk or egg substitutes.

Spinach and Mushroom Egg-Light Frittata

Number of Servings: Serves 6
***Ingredients*:**
- 3 cloves of garlic, minced
- 1 cup of chopped onion
- 1 teaspoon of olive oil
- ½ pound of fresh mushrooms, sliced
- ½ teaspoon of dried thyme
- 10 ounces of fresh spinach
- 1 tablespoon of water
- Egg substitute equivalent to 10 eggs

- 1 teaspoon of dehydrated dill or one tablespoon of freshly chopped dill
- ¼ teaspoon of black pepper
- ¼ cup of feta cheese (omit for a plant-based version)

Preparation Instructions:
1. Preheat the oven to 350°F (175°C).
2. In a 10- or 12-inch nonstick, ovenproof frying pan, sauté the garlic and onion in olive oil for about 5 minutes. Add the mushrooms and thyme, cooking for an additional 5 minutes. Remove the skillet from the stove.
3. Place the spinach in a separate saucepan with 1 tablespoon of water. Cover and cook until just wilted. Drain the spinach and let it cool in a colander. Squeeze out any excess liquid and chop the leaves.
4. In a large bowl, beat together the egg substitute, dill, and pepper. Add the blend of spinach and mushrooms along with the crumbled feta cheese.
5. Clean the pan and spray it liberally with cooking spray. Return the skillet to medium heat. When hot, pour in the egg mixture.
6. Place the saucepan in the oven, uncovered. Check the frittata after 10 minutes, then every 5 minutes thereafter, until the center is slightly firm. Avoid overcooking.

7. Once done, place a large serving platter over the saucepan and flip it over so the frittata falls onto the plate. Cut into six pieces and serve.

Dietitian's Tip:
This frittata uses an egg substitute instead of whole eggs to cut down on fat, cholesterol, and calories, making it a healthier choice. For added flavor, consider using roasted red bell peppers. To make this dish plant-based, omit the feta cheese or use a plant-based cheese alternative.

Smoky Bean and Mushroom Cornucopias

Number of Servings: Serves 6
Ingredients:
- 1 tablespoon canola oil
- 2 cloves fresh garlic, minced
- ½ cup diced yellow onion
- ½ cup chopped cremini mushrooms
- ¼ cup diced bell pepper
- 1 cup spinach, chopped
- 8 ounces of prepared black beans, thoroughly rinsed and drained
- 2 teaspoons chili powder
- 4 ounces fat-free sour cream (or a plant-based sour cream substitute)

- 1 teaspoon liquid smoke
- ¼ cup hot water (150-175°F)
- Six half-cut, six-inch diameter whole-wheat tortillas
- 2 teaspoons lime zest (optional, for garnish)

Preparation Instructions:
1. Preheat the oven to 375°F.
2. Place a spacious sauté pan on a medium flame, then introduce oil along with garlic. Cook the garlic for about 1 minute. Then, add the onion and cook until it begins to brown.
3. Add the mushrooms and cook for 2 minutes longer. Add the bell peppers and cook for 1 minute. Then, stir in the spinach, beans, and chili powder. Remove from heat after stirring well.
4. Let the mixture cool for 5 minutes, then fold in the sour cream and liquid smoke.
5. To assemble the cornucopias, lay out the tortilla halves on a cutting board and brush the cut edges lightly with hot water. Pinch together the two corners of each tortilla half and seal the edge to create the cornucopia shell. Arrange the shells on a parchment-lined baking tray.
6. Fill the tortillas with the bean and mushroom mixture. Place in the oven and cook for a duration of 20 to 25 minutes, or

until the internal temperature hits 165 degrees Fahrenheit.
7. Serve immediately, garnished with lime zest if desired, and accompanied by your favorite salsa.

Dietitian's Tip:
This dish is an excellent source of fiber, making it satisfying and beneficial for digestion. For those following a plant-based diet, simply omit the sour cream or use a plant-based alternative to make the recipe fully vegan.

Spring Vegetable Rice Noodles

Number of Servings: Serves 6
Ingredients:
- 1 package (8 ounces) rice noodles
- 1 tablespoon peanut oil
- 1 tablespoon sesame oil
- 1 tablespoon grated fresh ginger
- 2 garlic cloves, finely chopped
- 2 tablespoons reduced-sodium soy sauce
- 1 cup small broccoli florets
- 1 cup fresh bean sprouts
- 8 cherry tomatoes, halved
- 1 cup chopped fresh spinach
- 2 scallions, chopped
- Crushed red chili flakes (optional)

Preparation Instructions:
1. Pour water into a sizable pot until it is three-quarters full and heat until it reaches a rolling boil. Place the rice noodles in the boiling water and allow them to soften until they are just tender, which should take approximately 5 to 6 minutes, or follow the instructions specified on the packaging. Once cooked, drain the noodles and wash them thoroughly with cold water before setting them aside.
2. Warm the peanut and sesame oils in a large skillet or saucepan set over a medium flame. Introduce the ginger and garlic, sautéing them until they emit a pleasant aroma.
3. Add the soy sauce and broccoli into the pan, continuing to sauté over a medium setting for roughly 3 minutes.
4. Add the remaining vegetables (bean sprouts, cherry tomatoes, spinach, and scallions) and the cooked noodles, and toss until warmed through.
5. Portion out the noodles into heated dishes and, if preferred, garnish with a sprinkling of crushed red chili flakes.

Dietitian's Tip:
To limit the sodium in this stir-fry, the recipe uses reduced-sodium soy sauce. This dish is a great way

to enjoy a variety of vegetables, providing a wealth of nutrients and flavors.

Spinach, Chickpea, and Raisin Pasta

Number of Servings: Serves 6
Ingredients:
- Approximately 3 cups of uncooked farfalle pasta, weighing 8 ounces
- 2 tablespoons olive oil
- 4 garlic cloves, crushed
- ½ of a 19-ounce can of garbanzos (chickpeas), rinsed and drained
- ½ cup unsalted chicken broth (or vegetable broth for a vegetarian version)
- ½ cup golden raisins
- 4 cups fresh spinach, chopped
- 2 tablespoons grated Parmesan cheese (omit for a vegan version)
- Cracked black peppercorns, to taste

Preparation Instructions:
1. Pour water into a sizable pot, ensuring it reaches three-quarters of its capacity, and set it on high heat until it reaches a rolling boil.
2. Introduce the pasta into the boiling water, cooking it until it achieves an al dente texture, typically taking between 10 to 12

minutes, or follow the instructions specified on the pasta's packaging. After cooking, ensure the pasta is well-drained.
3. Proceed by warming the olive oil and garlic in a spacious frying pan over a medium flame.
4. Add the garbanzo beans and the broth, stirring the mixture until it is evenly heated.
5. Next, integrate the raisins and spinach into the contents of the frying pan. Continue to heat the mixture briefly, just until you observe the spinach beginning to wilt, which should take approximately 3 minutes. Avoid overcooking to preserve the nutrients in the spinach.
6. Divide the pasta among the plates. Top each serving with ⅙ of the sauce, sprinkle with 1 teaspoon of Parmesan cheese, and add peppercorns to taste. Serve immediately.

Dietitian's Tip:
The key to this recipe is to have the pasta and sauce done at the same time so that they don't overcook. This dish is a great opportunity for teamwork in the kitchen.

©Nancy K. Doctor

Tropical Mango Salsa Pizza

Number of Servings: Serves 4

Ingredients:
- 1 cup chopped red or green bell peppers
- ½ cup minced onion
- ½ cup chopped mango
- ½ cup pineapple tidbits
- 1 tablespoon lime juice
- ½ cup chopped fresh cilantro
- 1 12-inch prepared whole-grain pizza crust, purchased or made from a mix

Preparation Instructions:
1. Preheat the oven to 425°F (220°C). Lightly coat a 12-inch round pizza pan with cooking spray.
2. In a small bowl, mix the bell peppers, onions, mango, pineapple, lime juice, and cilantro. Set aside.
3. Roll out the dough and press it into the prepared pan. Bake the crust for about 15 minutes, until it starts to brown slightly.
4. Remove the crust from the oven and evenly spread the mango salsa over it. Return the pizza to the oven and bake until the toppings are hot and the crust is fully browned, about 5 to 10 minutes more.
5. Divide the pizza into eight equal portions and present it at once.

Nutrition Expert Advice:
To skin a mango, slice the fruit into two segments, circumventing the seed. Rest one segment flesh-side atop a chopping board and etch a grid pattern of ¼-inch squares into the pulp, ensuring not to slice through the outer layer. Invert the segment, push the squares outward and trim the chunks from the rind.

Classic Hummus

Number of Servings: Serves 14
Ingredients:
- 2 cans (16 ounces each) of reduced-sodium chickpeas, keep ¼ cup of the liquid and rinse and drain the rest
- 1 tablespoon of extra-virgin olive oil
- ¼ cup of lemon juice
- 2 garlic cloves, minced
- ¼ teaspoon of cracked black pepper
- ¼ teaspoon of paprika
- 3 tablespoons of tahini (sesame paste)
- 2 tablespoons of chopped Italian flat-leaf parsley

Preparation Instructions:
1. In a blender or food processor, purée the chickpeas until smooth.
2. Add the olive oil, lemon juice, garlic, pepper, paprika, tahini, and parsley to the puréed chickpeas. Blend well to combine.

3. Bit by bit, incorporate the set-aside chickpea liquid, dispensing it one tablespoon at a time until the hummus achieves a dense, spreadable texture. You may present it straightaway or, if preferred, seal it and store it in the refrigerator until it's time to serve.

Dietitian's Tip:
For a variation in taste, consider substituting white, butter, or lima beans for chickpeas and 1 teaspoon of toasted ground cumin seeds for the paprika. If you're following a gluten-free diet, ensure the tahini brand is gluten-free.

Grilled Pork Tenderloin Fajitas

Number of Servings: Serves 8
Ingredients:
- 1 teaspoon of ground cumin
- ½ teaspoon of oregano
- ½ teaspoon of paprika
- ¼ teaspoon of ground coriander
- ¼ teaspoon of garlic powder
- 1 pound of pork tenderloin, cut into strips (½ inch wide and 2 inches long)
- 1 small onion, sliced
- 8 warm whole-grain wheat tortillas, each approximately 8 inches across
- ½ cup of shredded sharp cheddar cheese
- 4 medium tomatoes, diced (about 3 cups)

- 4 cups of shredded lettuce
- 1 cup of salsa

Preparation Instructions:

1. Prepare a fire in a charcoal grill or heat a gas grill or broiler to medium-high (about 400°F).
2. In a small bowl, combine the cumin, oregano, paprika, coriander, and garlic powder. Dredge the pork strips in the seasoning mix, ensuring they are completely coated.
3. Place the seasoned pork strips and sliced onions in a cast-iron pan or grill basket. Grill or broil at medium-high heat, turning occasionally, until the pork is browned on all sides, approximately 5 minutes.
4. To assemble the fajitas, distribute an equal amount of pork strips and onions onto each tortilla. Top each with 1 tablespoon of cheese, 2 tablespoons of tomatoes, ½ cup of shredded lettuce, and 2 tablespoons of salsa.
5. Fold the sides of the tortilla over the filling, then roll up to close.

Dietitian's Tip:

Using pork tenderloin instead of traditional beef steak reduces the amount of saturated fat in these fajitas, making them a healthier choice. For an even healthier option, consider using a low-fat cheese alternative or omitting the cheese.

Zesty Fish Tacos with Tomatillo Salsa

Number of Servings: Serves 4

Ingredients:
- 12 ounces of whitefish, such as cod or tilapia
- Optional: Salt and pepper to taste
- 1½ cups of shredded Napa cabbage (about ¼ head)
- 1 teaspoon of cumin
- 2 teaspoons of paprika
- ½ teaspoon of chili powder
- ¼ cup of diced small yellow onion
- 2 tablespoons of minced cilantro (or parsley if preferred)
- 2 diced red Fresno peppers
- Zest and juice of 1 lime (½ teaspoon zest, 1 tablespoon juice)
- 4 tablespoons of tomatillo salsa
- 4 whole-wheat tortillas (6-inch diameter), lightly grilled or toasted

Preparation Instructions:
1. If desired, season the fish with salt and pepper. Bake the fish at 375°F for about 20 minutes, or until the internal temperature reaches 145°F. Alternatively, you can grill the fish.

2. In a mixing bowl, combine the shredded cabbage, cumin, paprika, chili powder, diced onion, minced cilantro (or parsley), diced Fresno peppers, lime zest, and lime juice. Toss to mix well.
3. Once the fish is cooked, flake it and distribute it evenly onto the tortillas.
4. Top the fish with the cabbage and salsa mixture.
5. Serve the tacos immediately.

Dietitian's Tip:

If cilantro isn't to your liking, parsley is a great alternative that doesn't compromise the flavor. This recipe is a healthy alternative to traditional beef tacos, offering a good balance of protein, fiber, and essential nutrients.

SALAD

Herb-Infused French Lentil Salad

Number of Servings: Serves 6
***Ingredients*:**
- 4 tablespoons of olive oil, divided
- ½ of a yellow onion, finely chopped
- A 4-inch piece of celery stalk, finely chopped
- A 4-inch piece of carrot peeled and finely chopped
- 3 cloves of garlic, minced
- 1 teaspoon of mustard seed
- 1 teaspoon of fennel seed
- 2 cups of vegetable or chicken stock (low sodium)
- ½ cup of water
- 1 cup of French green lentils, sorted, rinsed, and drained
- 1 tablespoon of fresh thyme or 1 teaspoon of dried thyme
- 1 bay leaf
- 1 tablespoon of sherry vinegar or red wine vinegar
- 1 tablespoon of Dijon mustard
- 2 tablespoons of fresh flat-leaf parsley, cut into strips

- ¼ teaspoon of freshly ground black pepper

Preparation Instructions:

1. In a large saucepan, warm 2 teaspoons of olive oil over medium heat. Add the chopped onion, celery, and carrot, sautéing until the vegetables soften, about 5 minutes.
2. Stir in the minced garlic, mustard seed, and fennel seed, cooking until the spices become fragrant, roughly 1 minute.
3. Pour in the stock, and water, and add the lentils, thyme, and bay leaf. Increase the heat to medium-high to bring the mixture to a boil, then reduce the heat to low. Partially cover and simmer until the lentils are tender yet firm, about 25 to 30 minutes.
4. Drain the lentils, saving the cooking liquid. Remove the lentils to a large bowl and discard the bay leaf.
5. For the dressing, mix the vinegar, Dijon mustard, and ¼ cup of the reserved cooking liquid in a small bowl. Discard any remaining liquid or save it for another use. Whisk in the remaining olive oil.
6. Add the dressing, parsley, and black pepper to the lentils. Toss gently to combine and evenly coat the lentils.
7. Serve the salad warm for the best flavor.

Dietitian's Tip:
French green lentils are preferred for their firm texture and nutty flavor, making them ideal for salads. If unavailable, brown lentils can be used but tend to be softer. This salad is high in fiber and protein, making it an excellent choice for those managing diabetes or following a renal diet.

Apple, Cranberry, and Walnut Salad

Ingredients:
- Red grapes, rinsed and halved
- Walnut halves, chopped
- Dried pomegranate-infused cranberries
- Celery, chopped
- Gala apples, cored and chopped
- Cranberry dressing (8 fluid ounces)

Directions:
1. Place halved grapes in a large mixing bowl.
2. Add chopped walnuts to the grapes.
3. Mix in the dried cranberries.
4. Add chopped celery to the mixture.
5. Incorporate the chopped apples.
6. Pour cranberry dressing over the mixture and stir well to ensure all ingredients are coated.
7. Chill the salad before serving.

Tips:
- For a variation, try using different types of apples or nuts.
- Ensure the cranberry dressing is low in sodium and sugar to maintain its kidney-friendly properties.

Tangy Pickled Onion and Herb Salad

Number of Servings: Serves 4
Ingredients:
- 2 large red onions, thinly sliced (approximately 2 cups)
- 4 spring onions (green onions), with tops, chopped
- ½ cup of cider vinegar
- 2 teaspoons of olive oil
- 2 tablespoons of sugar
- ½ cup of fresh cilantro, chopped
- 1 tablespoon of lime juice
- 4 lettuce leaves (for serving)

Preparation Instructions:
1. In a small mixing bowl, combine the thinly sliced red onions, chopped spring onions, cider vinegar, olive oil, and sugar. Stir the mixture well to ensure the onions are evenly coated with the vinegar and oil.

2. Cover the bowl and refrigerate the onion mixture for about 60 minutes to allow the flavors to meld and the onions to pickle slightly.
3. Just before serving, stir the chopped fresh cilantro into the chilled onion mixture. Sprinkle the lime juice over the top and give it one final mix.
4. To serve, place a lettuce leaf on each plate and mound an equal portion of the pickled onion salad on top of each leaf.

Dietitian's Tip:
This salad is a refreshing choice for summer and offers a tangy complement to grilled meats or as a vibrant topping for fish like tuna steaks. The combination of vinegar and lime juice not only adds flavor but also minimizes the need for added salt, making it a heart-healthy option.

Pear and Fennel Salad with Walnuts

Number of Servings: Serves 6
Ingredients:
- 6 cups of mixed salad greens
- One medium-sized bulb of fennel, neatly trimmed and finely sliced

- Two medium pears, with cores removed, cut into quarters and sliced thinly
- 2 tablespoons of grated Parmesan cheese (optional for a plant-based diet)
- ¼ cup of toasted walnuts, coarsely chopped
- 2 tablespoons of extra-virgin olive oil
- 3 tablespoons of balsamic vinegar
- Freshly ground black pepper, to taste

Preparation Instructions:

1. Begin by dividing the mixed salad greens evenly onto 6 plates.
2. Disperse the finely cut slices of fennel and pear across the bed of leafy greens.
3. If using, sprinkle the grated Parmesan cheese and the coarsely chopped toasted walnuts over the top of the salads.
4. Drizzle each salad with the extra-virgin olive oil and balsamic vinegar.
5. Season with freshly ground black pepper according to your taste preferences.
6. Serve the salads immediately to enjoy the fresh and crisp flavors.

Dietitian's Tip:

Fennel offers a unique, mild licorice flavor that compliments the sweetness of the pears and the crunchy texture of the walnuts. This salad offers a robust taste profile while being rich in essential nutrients. For those following a plant-based diet, you can easily omit the Parmesan cheese without losing the essence of the salad.

Chilled Shrimp and Apple Stuffed Tomatoes

Number of Servings: Serves 4
Ingredients:
- 1 tablespoon of water
- 1 cup of miniature shrimp, previously frozen and subsequently defrosted (equivalent to 48 pieces)
- 2 tablespoons of chopped red onion
- 2 medium apples, cored and cubed
- ¼ cup of lemon juice
- ½ cup of diced celery
- 1 tablespoon of chopped parsley
- 1 teaspoon of dried dill
- 4 teaspoons of horseradish
- ½ cup of fat-free mayonnaise
- Ground black pepper, to taste
- 4 large tomatoes, cored

Preparation Instructions:
1. Warm the water in a nonstick frying pan, setting the burner to a medium temperature. Add the thawed shrimp and chopped red onion. Sauté until the shrimp turns opaque and the onions are translucent approximately

5 to 7 minutes. Transfer the shrimp and onion mixture to a bowl, cover, and refrigerate until well-chilled.
2. In a small bowl, toss the cubed apples with lemon juice to coat evenly. Set aside.
3. In a large bowl, mix the diced celery, chopped parsley, dried dill, horseradish, and fat-free mayonnaise. Adjust seasoning by adding freshly ground black pepper according to your preference.
4. Stir the chilled shrimp mixture and the lemon-coated apples into the mayonnaise mixture. Refrigerate the combined salad for 45 to 60 minutes until well-chilled.
5. Just before serving, evenly divide and stuff the shrimp-apple salad into the cored tomatoes.

Dietitian's Tip:
This refreshing salad combines the sweetness of apples with the tanginess of lemon and horseradish, offering a delightful contrast of flavors. Shrimp provides a lean source of protein, making this dish a nutritious option for those managing diabetes or following a renal diet. For a plant-based alternative, omit the shrimp and increase the quantity of apples and celery.

©Nancy K. Doctor

Fresh Spinach and Mixed Berry Salad

Number of Servings: Serves 4
Ingredients:
Salad:
- 4 packed cups of fresh spinach, torn into bite-sized pieces
- 1 cup of fresh strawberries, sliced
- 1 cup of fresh or frozen blueberries
- 1 small sweet onion, thinly sliced
- ¼ cup of pecans, chopped and toasted

Salad Dressing:
- Two tablespoons of either distilled white vinegar or apple cider vinegar
- 2 tablespoons of balsamic vinegar
- 2 tablespoons of honey (or maple syrup for a plant-based option)
- 2 teaspoons of Dijon mustard
- 1 teaspoon of curry powder (optional)
- ⅛ teaspoon of pepper

Preparation Instructions:
1. In a large salad bowl, combine the spinach, strawberries, blueberries, onion, and pecans. Toss gently to mix.
2. For the dressing, in a jar with a tight-fitting lid, add the white wine vinegar, balsamic vinegar, honey (or maple syrup), Dijon

mustard, curry powder (if using), and pepper. Secure the lid and shake well until all the ingredients are well combined.
3. Just before serving, pour the dressing over the salad. Toss the salad again to ensure all the ingredients are evenly coated with the dressing.
4. Serve the salad immediately to enjoy its freshness and vibrant flavors.

Dietitian's Tip:
This vibrant salad isn't just visually appealing, it's also loaded with essential nutrients. Spinach and berries are excellent sources of vitamins and antioxidants, while pecans add a satisfying crunch and healthy fats. The homemade dressing is a healthier alternative to store-bought versions, allowing you to control the amount of sugar and sodium.

Honey-Dressed Warm Cabbage and Carrot Slaw

Number of Servings: Serves 6
Ingredients:
- 6 teaspoons of olive oil, divided
- 1 medium yellow onion, finely chopped (about ½ cup)
- 1 teaspoon of dry mustard

- One large-sized carrot, peeled, and cut into fine strips (approximately one cup)
- ½ head of Napa cabbage, cored and thinly sliced crosswise (about 5 cups)
- 3 tablespoons of cider vinegar
- 1 tablespoon of dark honey
- ¼ teaspoon of salt
- ¼ teaspoon of freshly ground black pepper
- ½ teaspoon of caraway seed
- 1 tablespoon of finely minced fresh Italian flat-leaf parsley

Preparation Instructions:

1. In a large nonstick sauté pan, heat 2 teaspoons of olive oil over medium-high heat until hot but not smoking. Add the chopped onion and dry mustard, sautéing until the onion is soft and lightly golden, about 6 minutes. Go ahead and move the chopped onion into a big mixing bowl.
2. Reduce the heat to medium and add another 2 teaspoons of olive oil to the pan. Add the julienned carrot, tossing and stirring constantly until the carrot is tender-crisp, about 3 minutes. Transfer the carrot to the bowl with the onion.
3. Add the remaining 2 teaspoons of olive oil to the pan over medium heat. Add the sliced cabbage, tossing and stirring constantly until the cabbage just begins to wilt, about 3

minutes. Quickly move the cabbage into the bowl where the rest of the veggies are hanging out.

4. Quickly add the cider vinegar and honey to the pan over medium heat, stirring until combined and bubbly and the honey is dissolved. Pour this warm dressing over the slaw in the bowl. Add the salt and pepper, and toss well to combine.
5. Garnish the slaw with caraway seed and chopped parsley. Serve the slaw warm.

Dietitian's Tip:
This slaw offers a twist on traditional coleslaw by serving it warm, which can enhance the flavors of the vegetables and dressing. Using olive oil and honey in the dressing provides a healthier alternative to mayonnaise-based dressings, contributing to heart health and managing blood sugar levels.

Tri-Color Tomato Basil Salad

Number of Servings: Serves 6
Ingredients:
For the Vinaigrette:
- Two tablespoons of either sherry vinegar or red wine vinegar
- 1 tablespoon of minced shallot
- 1 tablespoon of extra-virgin olive oil

- ¼ teaspoon of salt
- ⅛ teaspoon of freshly ground black pepper

For the Salad:
- 1½ cups of yellow pear tomatoes, halved
- 1½ cups of orange cherry tomatoes, halved
- 1½ cups of red cherry tomatoes, halved
- 4 large basil leaves, freshly picked, sliced into thin strips

Preparation Instructions:

1. To prepare the vinaigrette, in a small bowl, combine the vinegar and shallot. Let the mixture stand for 15 minutes to allow the flavors to meld. Then, whisk in the olive oil, salt, and pepper until the mixture is well blended.
2. In a large serving or salad bowl, gently toss together the halved yellow pear tomatoes, orange cherry tomatoes, and red cherry tomatoes.
3. Drizzle the prepared vinaigrette over the tomatoes. Add the basil ribbons and toss gently to ensure the tomatoes are evenly coated with the dressing.
4. Serve the salad immediately to enjoy the fresh and vibrant flavors.

Dietitian's Tip:

The colorful combination of yellow, orange, and red tomatoes not only makes this salad visually appealing but also provides a variety of antioxidants, including lycopene, which is known for its health benefits. The addition of fresh basil enhances the flavor profile, making this salad a perfect accompaniment to any meal.

Nourish to flourish. Even the smallest ingredient holds the power to heal in the kitchen. In life, balance is key. Let your meals be a testament to harmony.

©Nancy K. Doctor

SAUCE AND DRESSING

Sweetened Balsamic Dressing

Number of Servings: Serves 8

Ingredients:
- ½ cup of water
- 6 tablespoons of sugar
- ½ cup of dark balsamic vinegar
- 2 tablespoons of olive oil
- 4 cloves of garlic, minced
- ¼ teaspoon of kosher salt
- ¼ teaspoon of ground black pepper

Preparation Instructions:
1. Place a small saucepan over medium-low heat. Combine the water and sugar in the saucepan, stirring until the sugar begins to caramelize and turn a golden color.
2. Carefully add the balsamic vinegar, olive oil, minced garlic, kosher salt, and ground black pepper to the caramelized sugar. Be cautious as the mixture may splatter when the vinegar is added.
3. Remove the saucepan from the heat. Whisk the mixture thoroughly and allow it to cool. Once cooled, strain the dressing to remove the garlic pieces, discarding them.

4. The dressing is ready to be served immediately over your favorite salad. If you're not using it right away, store the dressing in a container. It will solidify when refrigerated, so gently warm it in the microwave or on the stove for a few seconds before use.

Dietitian's Tip:
This rich and sweet vinaigrette pairs exceptionally well with salads that contain tart elements, such as apples or dried cherries. The dressing's unique flavor profile can elevate a simple salad to a gourmet level. Remember, this dressing will solidify due to the sugar content when stored in the refrigerator, so warming it slightly will return it to a liquid state.

Creamy Greek Yogurt Ranch Dressing

Number of Servings: Serves 20
Ingredients:
- 2 cups of plain fat-free Greek yogurt
- ½ cup of low-fat mayonnaise
- 2 tablespoons of lemon juice
- 1 tablespoon of dried dill weed
- ½ tablespoon of onion powder
- ½ tablespoon of garlic powder

- ½ teaspoon of kosher salt
- ¼ teaspoon of black pepper

Preparation Instructions:
1. In a food processor, add the plain fat-free Greek yogurt, low-fat mayonnaise, lemon juice, dried dill weed, onion powder, garlic powder, kosher salt, and black pepper.
2. Process the mixture until all the ingredients are well combined and the dressing is smooth. Pause occasionally to scrape down the sides of the food processor bowl to ensure even mixing.
3. Once the dressing is thoroughly mixed, it can be served immediately. Alternatively, the dressing can be stored in a sealed plastic container in the refrigerator for up to 2 weeks.

Dietitian's Tip:
This healthier version of ranch dressing uses fat-free Greek yogurt as a base, providing a creamy texture without the added calories and fats found in traditional ranch dressings. It's a versatile dressing that can be used on salads, as a dip for vegetables, or as a condiment for grilled meats. For those on a Diabetic Renal Diet, this dressing offers a flavorful option without compromising dietary restrictions.

©Nancy K. Doctor

Honeyed Peach Puree

Number of Servings: Serves 4
Ingredients:
- One can (15 ounces) of peach halves without added sugar, with the liquid removed
- 2 tablespoons of honey
- ½ teaspoon of cinnamon

Preparation Instructions:
1. In a large mixing bowl, combine the drained peach halves, honey, and cinnamon.
2. Using a fork or a potato masher, mash the ingredients together until the mixture reaches the consistency of a chunky applesauce. For a smoother texture, you could also use a blender or food processor.
3. The Honeyed Peach Puree can be served immediately or stored in a covered container in the refrigerator until ready to use.

Dietitian's Tip:
This versatile peach spread is an excellent way to add natural sweetness and flavor to various dishes. It pairs wonderfully with breakfast items like pancakes or French toast and can also complement savory dishes such as roasted chicken or pork. For those managing diabetes, remember to account for the honey in your total carbohydrate intake. Alternatives like pears, apricots, plums, or

nectarines can also be used in place of peaches to vary the flavor.

Nutty Chickpea Spread

Number of Servings: Serves 16
Ingredients:
- 2 cups of garbanzo beans (chickpeas)
- 1 cup of water
- ½ cup of powdered peanut butter
- ¼ cup of natural peanut butter
- 2 tablespoons of brown sugar
- 1 teaspoon of vanilla extract

Preparation Instructions:
1. Combine the garbanzo beans, water, powdered peanut butter, natural peanut butter, brown sugar, and vanilla extract in a food processor.
2. Blend the mixture until it achieves a smooth and creamy consistency. You may need to pause and scrape down the sides of the food processor bowl to ensure all ingredients are well incorporated.
3. Once the mixture is thoroughly blended, transfer the hummus to a container and refrigerate. The hummus can be stored in the refrigerator for up to 1 week.

Dietitian's Tip:
This unique twist on traditional hummus incorporates peanut butter for a creamy texture and a nutty flavor profile. It's a versatile spread that can be enjoyed with fresh fruit slices, such as apples or celery, making it a perfect snack for those managing diabetes or following a renal diet. The addition of powdered peanut butter reduces the fat content without sacrificing flavor.

Every meal is a step on the journey to your well-being. Choose paths that lead to a vibrant and healthy kidney health destination.

SIDE DISHES

Refreshing Sugar-Free Coleslaw

Cooking Time: 10 mins | Serving Size: 2 servings

Ingredients:
- 1 cup red cabbage, thinly sliced
- 1 cup green cabbage, thinly sliced
- 1 medium radish, grated
- ½ tsp celery seed
- ¼ cup plain yogurt (1-2% M.F.)
- 2 tsp apple cider vinegar
- 1 tsp lemon juice
- 1 packet of stevia sweetener, powder
- ¼ tsp salt
- A dash of black pepper

Directions:
1. In a medium bowl, mix the red cabbage, green cabbage, radish, and celery seed.
2. In a separate small bowl, whisk together the yogurt, apple cider vinegar, lemon juice, stevia, salt, and pepper until well combined.
3. Pour the yogurt dressing over the cabbage mixture and toss to coat evenly.

Tips:
- Modify the quantity of stevia to suit your desired level of sweetness.

- This coleslaw can be refrigerated for a few hours before serving to enhance the flavors.

Quick and Nutritious Tuna Salad

Cooking Time: 5 minutes | Serving Size: 1 serving

Ingredients:
- 1 can albacore tuna, drained
- ¼ stalk celery, diced
- ½ medium red bell pepper, sliced
- 1 artichoke heart, quartered
- ½ cup cucumber, peeled and sliced
- 1 small pear, chopped
- ½ tablespoon green onion
- ¼ small carrot, chopped
- 3 cups romaine lettuce or mixed greens
- 1 tablespoon extra virgin olive oil
- 1 tablespoon balsamic vinegar

Directions:
1. In a bowl, mix lettuce and vegetables. Drizzle with olive oil and balsamic vinegar as dressing.
2. Top the salad with drained tuna.
3. Adjust the seasoning by adding salt and pepper according to your preference.

Tips:

- Feel free to substitute any of the vegetables with your favorites or what's available in season.
- For a lower-sodium version, choose low-sodium canned tuna.

Simple Cauliflower Rice

Cooking Time: 10 minutes | Serving Size: 1 serving

Ingredients:
- 1 medium head of cauliflower
- 1 tablespoon of premium extra virgin olive oil or clarified butter (ghee)
- A pinch of sea salt

Directions:
1. Cut the cauliflower into large florets.
2. Use a food processor with a shredding blade or pulse with a chopping blade to 'rice' the cauliflower. Alternatively, grate it by hand on a box grater.
3. Heat olive oil in a large frying pan over medium heat. Add the cauliflower rice and sauté until just cooked through, about 5 minutes.

Tips:
- *For added flavor, you can mix in herbs or spices.*

- Be careful not to overcook the cauliflower to maintain a rice-like texture.

Kale and Broccoli Power Bowl

Cooking Time: 8 minutes | Serving Size: 1 serving

Ingredients:
- 1½ cups chopped kale
- ½ cup chopped raw broccoli
- ½ avocado, cubed
- 1 tsp lemon juice (to taste)
- 1 tsp extra virgin olive oil
- A pinch of salt (to taste)
- 2 tbsp hulled hemp seeds (optional)

Directions:
1. Heat 2 inches of water in a large pot with a steamer basket. Once boiling, reduce the heat and add kale and broccoli. Steam for 3 minutes, then transfer to a bowl.
2. Add avocado, lemon juice, olive oil, salt, and hemp seeds (if using).
3. Toss gently to combine. Adjust lemon juice, oil, or salt as needed.

Tips:
- Steaming preserves most of the nutrients in the greens.
- Adjust the amount of lemon juice and olive oil to suit your taste preferences.

Sweet Honey and Sage Glazed Carrots

Servings: 4 servings.

Ingredients:
- Carrots, sliced, 2 cups
- Butter, 2 teaspoons
- Honey, 2 tablespoons
- Fresh sage, chopped, 1 tablespoon
- Ground black pepper, ¼ teaspoon
- Salt, ⅛ teaspoon

Preparation Instructions:
1. Begin by boiling a medium-sized pot of water. Once boiling, add the sliced carrots and cook for about 5 minutes until they are tender enough to be pierced with a fork.
2. Drain the water from the carrots and put them to one side.
3. Heat a medium sauté pan over medium heat and melt the butter in it. Once the butter has melted and the pan is hot, add the boiled carrots along with the honey, chopped sage, black pepper, and salt.
4. Sauté the mixture for approximately 3 minutes, stirring often to ensure the carrots are evenly coated with the honey and sage mixture. Once done, remove from heat and the dish is ready to serve.

Dietitian's Tip:
To ensure the carrots have reached the perfect level of tenderness, test a slice by boiling it separately. This helps in achieving the ideal texture for the dish.

Easy Fried Rice

Serving size: 4 servings | Prep time: 25 minutes | Total time: 25 minutes

Ingredients:
- 1 teaspoon plus 2 tablespoons peanut or canola oil, divided
- 2 large eggs, beaten
- 3 scallions, thinly sliced
- 2 teaspoons grated fresh ginger
- 2 teaspoons minced garlic
- 2 cups mixed frozen vegetables (thawed)
- 2 cups cold cooked brown rice
- 2½ tablespoons reduced-sodium soy sauce

Directions:
1. Begin by heating a teaspoon of oil in a sizable carbon-steel wok or a large, sturdy frying pan over a high flame. Crack the eggs into the pan and let them fry undisturbed until they're set on one side, which should take about half a minute.
2. Flip them over and give them another 15 seconds or so, just until they're cooked all

the way through. Then, slide them onto a chopping board and chop them into bite-sized, half-inch chunks.
3. Now, it's time to drizzle in a tablespoon of oil to the same wok. Toss in the scallions, ginger, and garlic, and give them a quick stir-fry until the scallions become soft and fragrant, which should be no more than 30 seconds.
4. Next, add your mix of veggies and stir-fry them until they're crisp-tender, which might take anywhere from 2 to 4 minutes. Once they're done, scoop everything out of the wok and onto a big plate.
5. For the final touch, pour the last tablespoon of oil into the wok. Tumble in the rice and stir it around until it's thoroughly heated, which should take about 1 to 2 minutes. Keep stirring and turning the rice from the bottom up to the top to make sure each grain is nicely coated with oil and heated evenly.
6. Return the vegetables and eggs to the wok; add soy sauce and stir until well combined.

Tips:
If you're managing celiac disease or sensitive to gluten, always grab soy sauce that's marked "gluten-free." Some soy sauces sneak in wheat or gluten-packed additives for sweetness and flavor, so it's best to check the label to stay safe.

Savory Roasted Asparagus and Mushroom Medley Stew

Total Cooking Time: 35 minutes
Ingredients:
- Asparagus spears
- Olive oil for spraying
- Dried mushrooms, reconstituted in hot water
- Celery, diced
- Carrots, diced
- Onions, diced
- Fennel, diced
- Marsala wine, thyme, ground cayenne, minced sage, and finely diced parsley
- Bay leaf
- Garlic powder, onion powder
- Vegetable stock
- Pine nuts for garnish

Directions:
1. Preheat the oven to 400°F. Prepare asparagus by washing and trimming the tough ends.
2. Arrange asparagus in a single layer on a baking sheet and lightly spray with olive oil. Bake for 10 minutes, then cool and cut into 1-inch pieces.
3. Reconstitute dried mushrooms in hot water.

4. In a saucepan, heat olive oil and sauté celery, carrots, onions, and fennel until onions are translucent. Add herbs, spices, Marsala wine, bay leaf, garlic, and onion powders, and stir for another minute.
5. Add vegetable stock and the liquid from the mushrooms. Heat until it gently simmers and continue cooking for fifteen minutes.
6. Place roasted asparagus in the serving dish, pour the stew over, and sprinkle with pine nuts.

Tips:
- For a more robust flavor, roast the mushrooms along with the asparagus.
- Serve with a side of whole-grain bread for a complete meal.

Strawberry Fruit Salad

Serves 8 (1 serving = ¾ cup) | Prep time: 10 mins | Total time: 40 minutes

Ingredients:
- 2 tablespoons honey
- 2 tablespoons lemon juice
- Six cups of fresh strawberries with their hulls removed, sliced into halves or quarters for the larger berries
- 2 cups fresh blackberries
- ¼ cup finely chopped fresh mint

Directions:
1. In a sizable bowl, combine honey and lemon juice by whisking them together.
2. Add both strawberries and blackberries to the mixture, carefully folding them in to ensure an even coating.
3. Allow the fruit to marinate for a minimum of 30 minutes, extending up to an hour for optimal flavor infusion.

Cobb Salad with Dijon Dressing

Serving size: 4 servings | Prep time: 40 minutes | Total time: 40 minutes

Ingredients:
- 3 tablespoons white-wine vinegar
- 2 tablespoons finely minced shallot
- 1 tablespoon Dijon mustard
- 1 teaspoon freshly ground pepper
- ¼ teaspoon salt
- 3 tablespoons extra-virgin olive oil
- 10 cups mixed salad greens
- 8 ounces of finely shredded, pre-cooked chicken breast meat, equivalent to one large breast (half)
- 2 large eggs, hard-boiled, peeled and chopped
- 2 medium tomatoes, diced
- 1 large cucumber, seeded and sliced

- 1 avocado, diced
- 2 slices cooked bacon, crumbled
- ½ cup crumbled blue cheese, (optional)

Directions:
1. In a compact bowl, blend vinegar, shallot, and mustard, along with a pinch of salt and pepper by whisking them thoroughly to ensure they are well combined. Whisk in oil until combined.
2. Place salad greens in a large bowl. Add half of the dressing and toss to coat.
3. Divide the greens among 4 plates. Go ahead and evenly distribute the chicken, egg, tomatoes, cucumber, avocado, bacon, and blue cheese (if you're tossing that in) over the bed of lettuce. Then give the salads a good drizzle with the leftover dressing.

Tips:
If you're looking to poach some chicken breasts, just grab a medium-sized skillet or pot and pop in your boneless, skinless chicken breasts. Pour in enough water to cover them and toss in a pinch of salt. Crank up the heat until it starts boiling, then slap a lid on it, turn the heat down to low, and let it simmer nice and easy. You're aiming for the chicken to be thoroughly cooked and not pink in the middle, which should take about 10 to 15 minutes. Once it's done, grab a couple of forks and shred that chicken into nice, long strips.

©Nancy K. Doctor

Quick Pickled Vegetables

Prep Time: 5 minutes | Cook Time: 30 minutes | Servings: 2¼ cup

Ingredients:
- ½ cup vinegar
- 2 Tbsp sugar
- 1 pinch salt
- ½ cup of your favorite veggie thinly sliced

Instructions:
1. Start by mixing vinegar, sugar, and a pinch of salt in a tiny pot.
2. Warm it up just until it starts to bubble gently. Keep stirring for around a minute or so, just until you see the sugar and salt melt away completely.
3. Now, go ahead and drizzle that tangy blend right over your veggies. Give them a good half-hour to soak it all in, or if you've got time, let them marinate for a full day.
4. Drain vegetables and enjoy!

Notes:
- *My favorite veggies to pickle are carrots, shallots, onions, carrots, cabbage, daikon, and jicama.*
- *Add marinated vegetables to infuse a MASSIVE burst of taste into a variety of dishes. Try them on sandwiches, salads, or tacos. I promise you will get addicted!*

©Nancy K. Doctor

Flavourful Lean Country Sausage

Servings: 6 servings
Ingredients:
- Lean ground pork loin, ½ pound
- Lean ground turkey breast, ½ pound
- Sugar, 1 teaspoon
- Dry mustard, 1 teaspoon
- Onion powder, 1 teaspoon
- Sage, 1 teaspoon
- Ground black pepper, 1 teaspoon
- Red pepper flakes (optional), ½ teaspoon

Preparation Instructions:
1. In a sizable bowl, combine the ground pork loin, ground turkey breast, sugar, dry mustard, onion powder, sage, black pepper, and optional red pepper flakes thoroughly.
2. Go ahead and form the mix into a dozen patties, all about the same size.
3. Coat a large nonstick frying pan with cooking spray and warm it over medium heat. Place the patties in the pan, cover, and cook until they are nicely browned and the juices run clear, which should take about 5 minutes per side. For those who prefer to use a thermometer, ensure the internal

temperature reaches 165°F (74°C) before removing from the heat.
4. Once cooked, transfer the patties to a serving dish and serve them hot.

Dietitian's Tip:
For those who prefer a milder taste, you can substitute the sage, black pepper, and red pepper flakes with 1 teaspoon of rosemary. Alternatively, for an Italian twist, replace the sage and red pepper flakes with 1 teaspoon of basil and ½ teaspoon of fennel. This allows you to adjust the flavor profile of the sausages to suit your taste preferences or dietary needs.

Golden Lemon Almond Rice

Servings: 8 servings
Ingredients:
- Slivered almonds (coarsely chopped), ½ cup
- Uncooked brown rice, 1 cup
- Unsalted chicken broth (or vegetable stock for a plant-based version), 1¾ cups
- Lemon juice, 3 tablespoons
- Lemon zest, 2 teaspoons
- Chopped onions, ¼ cup
- Ground cinnamon, ½ teaspoon
- Ground nutmeg, ¼ teaspoon
- Trans-free margarine, 1 tablespoon
- Water, ⅓ cup

- Golden raisins, ½ cup
- Frozen peas, ½ cup
- Honey, 2 tablespoons

Preparation Instructions:

1. Preheat your oven to 325°F (163°C) and lightly grease a baking sheet with cooking spray.
2. Spread the almonds on the prepared baking sheet and toast in the oven until they are golden brown and aromatic, about 10 minutes. Once done, immediately transfer them to a plate to cool.
3. In a medium saucepan over medium heat, combine the rice, chicken broth (or vegetable stock), lemon juice, lemon zest, onions, cinnamon, nutmeg, and margarine. Cover the saucepan and let it simmer, stirring occasionally, for about 30 minutes or until the rice has absorbed all the liquid.
4. In a separate, smaller saucepan, bring the water and raisins to a simmer. Cover and let it cook for 5 minutes, then add the peas and cook for an additional minute.
5. Combine the raisin and pea mixture with the rice, continuing to simmer until all the liquid is absorbed, which should take another 15 to 20 minutes.
6. Once fully cooked, fluff the rice mixture with a fork, transfer it to a serving dish, and

top with the toasted almonds. Drizzle honey over the dish before serving.

Dietitian's Tip:

Brown rice is chosen for this recipe due to its higher fiber, vitamin, and mineral content compared to white rice, making it a healthier choice. For a plant-based version, simply use vegetable stock instead of chicken broth.

Quick Roasted Green Beans

Servings: serves 4

Ingredients:
- Green beans, cleaned and trimmed, 2 cups
- Cherry tomatoes, about 20, 1 cup
- Minced garlic, 1 tablespoon
- Olive oil, 2 teaspoons
- Dried basil, 1 teaspoon
- Dried oregano, 1 teaspoon
- Onion powder, 1 teaspoon
- Salt, ½ teaspoon
- Pepper, ½ teaspoon

Preparation Instructions:
1. Preheat your oven to 400°F (204°C) and lightly oil a baking sheet.
2. In a medium-sized bowl, toss together the green beans, cherry tomatoes, garlic, olive oil, basil, oregano, onion powder, salt, and

pepper until the beans and tomatoes are well-coated with the oil and herbs.
3. Spread the green bean mixture out on the prepared baking sheet in a single layer.
4. Roast in the preheated oven for 10 to 15 minutes, stirring them after 10 minutes to ensure even cooking.

Dietitian's Tip:
If you prefer your green beans to be more tender, consider blanching them in boiling water for about 30 seconds before mixing them with the tomatoes and herbs. This extra step helps to soften the beans slightly before they go into the oven, enhancing their texture and flavor.

Delicious Spiced Buckwheat Pilaf

Servings: serve 6
<u>Ingredients:</u>
- Olive oil, 1 tablespoon
- Yellow onion, chopped, about 1 cup
- Buckwheat groats, 1 cup
- Garlic cloves, minced, 3
- Cumin seed, ½ teaspoon
- Mustard seed, ½ teaspoon
- Ground cardamom, ¼ teaspoon
- Unsalted vegetable stock or broth, 2 cups

- Tomato, peeled, seeded, and diced, about 1 cup
- Salt, ¼ teaspoon
- Fresh cilantro (coriander), chopped, 2 tablespoons

Preparation Instructions:

1. Initiate the cooking process by warming the olive oil in a saucepan on a medium flame. Add the chopped onion and sauté until it becomes soft and translucent, which should take about 4 minutes.
2. To the saucepan, add the buckwheat groats, minced garlic, cumin seed, mustard seed, and cardamom. Continue to sauté, stirring constantly, for about 3 minutes or until the spices become fragrant and the buckwheat is slightly toasted.
3. Pour the vegetable stock or broth into the saucepan carefully. Bring the mixture to a boil, then reduce the heat to medium-low, cover, and let it simmer until all the liquid has been absorbed for about 10 minutes.
4. After removing the saucepan from the heat, let it stand covered for an additional 2 minutes.
5. Stir in the diced tomato and salt. Move the pilaf to a serving bowl and garnish with the chopped cilantro before serving.

Dietitian's Tip:

Buckwheat groats, despite their name, are not related to wheat and are a gluten-free grain. They provide an abundant supply of dietary fiber, essential vitamins, and minerals. This pilaf, seasoned with fresh herbs and aromatic spices, offers a nutritious and flavorful alternative to traditional rice dishes.

Nutritious Tangy Green Beans

Servings: serve 10.
Ingredients:
- Green beans (fresh, frozen, or canned), 1½ pounds
- Sweet red bell peppers, diced, ⅓ cup
- For the Dressing:
- Olive oil or canola oil, 4½ teaspoons
- Water, 4½ teaspoons
- Vinegar, 1½ teaspoons
- Mustard, 1½ teaspoons
- Salt, ¼ teaspoon
- Pepper, ¼ teaspoon
- Garlic powder, ⅛ teaspoon

Preparation Instructions:
- Using a steamer basket over boiling water, steam the green beans and red peppers until they are crisp-tender.

- In a small bowl, whisk together the olive oil (or canola oil), water, vinegar, mustard, salt, pepper, and garlic powder to create the dressing.
- Once the beans and peppers are steamed to your liking, transfer them to a serving bowl.
- Pour the prepared dressing over the beans and peppers, and stir well to ensure they are evenly coated with the tangy mixture.
- Use the stock immediately, or store it in the refrigerator for up to 2 days. For longer storage, freeze the stock in airtight containers for up to 3 months.

Dietitian's Tip:
Creating your chicken stock at home is an effective way to control sodium levels, enhancing your dishes with natural flavors without the added salt found in many commercial broths. Browning the ingredients before simmering not only adds depth to the color but also enriches the stock with a complex flavor profile.

Hearty Vegetable Barley and Mushroom Soup

Servings: This recipe serves 9
Ingredients:
- Canola oil, 1 tablespoon

- Chopped onions, 1½ cups
- Sliced mushrooms, 1 cup
- Chopped carrots, ¾ cup
- Dried thyme, 1 teaspoon
- Black pepper, ⅛ teaspoon
- Chopped garlic, ½ teaspoon
- Vegetable stock, 8 cups
- Pearl barley, ¾ cup
- Dry sherry, 3 ounces (optional, can be replaced with extra broth)
- Small potato, chopped, ½
- Thinly sliced green onions, ¼ cup

Preparation Instructions:

1. In a large stockpot, warm the canola oil over medium-high heat. Add the onions, mushrooms, carrots, thyme, pepper, and garlic. Keep cooking the onions, stirring them around, until they turn nice and clear, which should take around five minutes or so.
2. Pour in the vegetable stock and add the barley. Bring the mixture to a boil, then lower the heat and simmer for approximately 20 minutes, or until the barley is tender.
3. Stir in the sherry (if using) and the chopped potato. Continue simmering until the potato is fully cooked, about 15 minutes.
4. Garnish the soup with sliced green onions before serving.

Dietitian's Tip:
This soup is a fantastic option for utilizing leftover vegetables in your fridge. If you have pre-cooked barley, add it towards the end of the cooking process, just long enough to warm it through. The sherry adds a depth of flavor but can be omitted or substituted with additional broth to suit your taste preferences or dietary needs.

Harness the power of your kitchen with different delicious and nutritious flavors to create a potion for health and happiness.

SNACKS

Almond Essence Cookies

**Prep Time: 30 minutes | Cooking Time: 15 minutes |
Serving Size: 3 cookies**

Ingredients:
- 1 cup of softened margarine
- 1 cup of sugar
- 1 large egg
- 3 cups of all-purpose flour
- 1 teaspoon of baking soda
- 1 teaspoon of almond extract

Instructions:
1. Preheat your oven to 400°F (200°C). In a medium-sized mixing bowl, cream together the softened margarine and sugar until smooth.
2. Crack the egg into the mixture and beat well to incorporate.
3. Sift together the flour and baking soda, then gradually add to the creamed mixture, mixing until just combined.
4. Stir in the almond extract, ensuring the dough is well-blended.
5. Roll the dough into balls, roughly ¾ inch in diameter. Place the balls on a baking sheet

and gently press a small indentation into the center of each cookie.
6. Place the cookies in the oven, which has been preheated, and allow them to cook for a duration of 10 to 12 minutes. They should be removed once the perimeters exhibit a pale golden-brown hue.

Spicy Cream Cheese Tortilla Rolls

Prep Time: 30 mins | Cooking Time: 10 mins | Serving Size: 3 pieces per serving

Ingredients:
- 5 large white tortillas
- 250g (1 package) cream cheese, softened
- ½ cup red bell peppers, finely chopped
- ½ cup green bell peppers, finely chopped
- ½ cup green onions, finely chopped
- ¼ cup jalapeños, finely chopped (optional for extra heat)
- ¼ cup bread crumbs, for added texture

Instructions:
1. Start the cooking by setting your oven to a temperature of 400 degrees Fahrenheit, which is equivalent to 200 degrees Celsius. This ensures the oven is ready by the time you finish preparing the antojitos.

2. Prepare the vegetables by finely chopping the red and green bell peppers, green onions, and jalapeños (if using). The fine chop will help distribute the flavors evenly throughout the cream cheese mixture.
3. In a large mixing bowl, combine the softened cream cheese with the chopped vegetables. Mix until the vegetables are fully incorporated into the cream cheese, creating a colorful and flavorful spread.
4. Lay out the tortillas on a clean work surface. Spread an even layer of the cream cheese mixture onto each tortilla, reaching close to the edges to ensure every bite is filled with flavor.
5. Carefully roll up the tortillas tightly to ensure the filling stays inside. Once rolled, use a sharp knife to cut each tortilla roll into six equal pieces. This will make them easier to handle and serve.
6. Arrange the cut tortilla rolls on a baking sheet, leaving some space between each piece. If you have bread crumbs, sprinkle them lightly over the tops of the rolls for an extra crunch.
7. Bake in the preheated oven for 7 to 10 minutes, or until the tops of the tortilla rolls are golden brown and the filling is heated through.

8. Take out of the oven and permit to cool for a short period before serving. These can be served as a delicious and spicy snack or as a side dish with your favorite Mexican meals.

Almond-Infused Pear Parfait

Total Time: Approx. 15 mins (plus chilling time)
Ingredients:
- Rice milk
- Flour
- Sugar
- Vanilla extract
- Almond extract
- Pears (specific amount not provided in the original recipe)

Directions:
1. Heat rice milk in a microwaveable bowl for 5 minutes on high.
2. Mix flour and sugar, then gradually add hot rice milk to form a smooth paste.
3. Return the mixture to the hot rice milk, stirring continuously.
4. Microwave the mixture for 1 minute and 30 seconds on high, then stir again.
5. Cook for an additional minute on high.
6. Remove from the microwave, add vanilla and almond extracts.

7. Pour into a shallow dish and refrigerate until chilled.
8. The mixture can be prepared up to 2 days in advance.
9. Serve chilled with layers of sliced pears.

Tips:
- For added texture, top with slivered almonds or a sprinkle of cinnamon.
- Substitute pears with other renal-friendly fruits like berries or apples.

DINNER RECIPES

Gingered Cranberry Chicken Delight

Prep Time: 45 mins | Cooking Time: 3 hours | Serving Size: 1½ cups

Ingredients:
- 2 cups of cranberry juice cocktail
- ½ cup of sweetened, dried cranberries
- 1 teaspoon of freshly grated ginger
- 1 clove of garlic, minced
- 1½ pounds of chicken thighs or breasts, bone-in, with skin removed
- 2 tablespoons of finely diced shallots
- 1 tablespoon of unsalted butter

- ½ cup of julienned carrots
- 2 tablespoons of fresh chives, finely chopped, for garnish

Instructions:
1. In a large mixing bowl, combine the cranberry juice, dried cranberries, grated ginger, and minced garlic. Stir well to blend.
2. Place the chicken pieces into the mixture, ensuring they are fully submerged. Cover the bowl and allow the chicken to marinate in the refrigerator for 1 to 2 hours.
3. After marinating, remove the chicken from the bowl, season with salt and pepper to taste, and set aside the marinade for later use.
4. Using a medium-sized saucepan, melt the butter over medium heat. Next, add your diced shallots and cook them until they become translucent.
5. Add the marinade that was set aside earlier into the saucepan and heat it until it reaches a boiling point. Reduce the heat to low and let it simmer for 15 minutes, allowing the sauce to reduce by half. Add the julienned carrots during the last 5 minutes of cooking.
6. Grill the marinated chicken over medium-high heat for 4 to 6 minutes on each side, or until the chicken is fully cooked and the juices run clear when pierced with a

fork. Make sure the inside temperature hits 165 degrees Fahrenheit, which is about 74 degrees Celsius, to be safe.
7. Arrange the grilled chicken on a serving platter. Drizzle the reduced marinade over the chicken and garnish with chopped chives.
8. Serve the chicken accompanied by seasonal vegetables and a whole grain side, such as brown rice or quinoa, for a balanced meal.

Zesty Lemon Thyme Tuna Pasta Salad

Prep Time: 30 minutes | Cooking Time: 15 minutes
Ingredients:
- 2 tablespoons dried thyme
- 4 teaspoons chopped chives
- 4 oz ziti pasta, dry
- 1 pouch (about 2.6 oz) low sodium Albacore White Tuna in Water, drained
- ⅛ teaspoon ground black pepper
- 1 teaspoon canola oil
- ⅛ teaspoon garlic powder (adjusted from "garlic" for clarity)
- 1½ teaspoon Dijon mustard
- ⅛ teaspoon dry mustard

- 2 tablespoons lemon juice

Preparation:
1. Begin by cooking the ziti pasta according to the package directions. Once cooked, rinse under cold water to cool and then drain thoroughly.
2. In a large mixing bowl, combine the cooked pasta, drained tuna, chopped chives, and dried thyme. Toss these ingredients gently to distribute the herbs and tuna evenly throughout the pasta.
3. For the dressing, whisk together the canola oil, garlic powder, Dijon mustard, dry mustard, lemon juice, and ground black pepper in a separate bowl until well combined. This mixture will create a tangy and flavorful dressing that complements the tuna and pasta perfectly.
4. Pour the dressing over the pasta and tuna mixture, tossing well to ensure every piece is coated with the dressing. The lemon juice and herbs will give the salad a fresh and vibrant flavor.
5. Serve the pasta salad garnished with a fresh sprig of lemon thyme (if available) or additional chopped chives for an extra touch of freshness and color.

©Nancy K. Doctor

Mexican-Inspired Turkey and Rice Stuffed Peppers

Prep Time: 30 minutes | Cooking Time: 1 hr | Serving Size: ½ stuffed pepper per serving

Ingredients:
- 3 red bell peppers, halved lengthwise and seeds removed
- ½ cup cooked brown rice
- 1 pound lean ground turkey (93% lean/7% fat)
- ½ cup plus 3 tablespoons fresh salsa, divided
- ½ cup onion, finely chopped
- 1 large egg
- 1 tablespoon chili powder
- ½ teaspoon black pepper
- 3 tablespoons cilantro, finely chopped
- Non-stick cooking spray
- 2 tablespoons water

Instructions:
1. Preheat your oven to 350°F (175°C). Prepare a baking dish by lightly spraying it with non-stick cooking spray.
2. Prepare the bell peppers by washing them, cutting them in half lengthwise, and removing the stems and inner membranes. Set the prepared pepper halves aside.

3. In a large bowl, mix the cooked brown rice, ground turkey, ½ cup of fresh salsa, chopped onion, egg, chili powder, black pepper, and chopped cilantro until well combined. This mixture will be the filling for your peppers.
4. Divide the turkey and rice mixture evenly among the six bell pepper halves, stuffing them generously.
5. Place the stuffed peppers cut-side up in the prepared baking dish. Pour 2 tablespoons of water into the bottom of the dish to help steam the peppers while they bake, keeping them moist.
6. Wrap the baking dish snugly in foil and pop it in your already hot oven. Let it cook for a solid 45 minutes.
7. After 45 minutes, remove the foil and spoon 1½ teaspoons of the remaining fresh salsa over each pepper half. Return the dish to the oven, uncovered, and bake for an additional 15 minutes, or until the peppers are tender and the filling is cooked through.
8. Serve and enjoy the warmth of the filled peppers, and should you desire, enhance their taste with an additional dash of cilantro.

Homemade Chicken Pad Thai

Prep Time: 30 minutes, Cooking Time: 55 minutes
Ingredients:
- 1 pound rice noodles (preferably low-sodium)
- ¼ cup vegetable oil
- 1 cup cooked chicken, thinly sliced
- 1 tablespoon minced garlic
- 4 green onions, sliced on the diagonal
- 1 chili pepper, finely diced
- 1 egg, lightly beaten
- ⅔ cup homemade or store-bought Pad Thai Sauce
- 1 lime, cut into wedges
- ⅛ cup cilantro, roughly chopped

Preparation:
1. Begin by soaking the rice noodles in warm water for about 40 minutes, or until they are soft but not fully cooked. Pour out the water from the noodles and keep them to one side.
2. While the noodles are soaking, cook the chicken if it is not already prepared. Once cooked, slice it into thin strips.
3. Prepare the Pad Thai Sauce according to your recipe or use a pre-made sauce. If made from scratch, typical ingredients include tamarind paste, fish sauce (or a vegetarian

alternative), sugar, and lime juice, adjusted to taste.
4. Warm the vegetable oil in a large skillet or wok over medium-high heat. Add the minced garlic, diced chili pepper, and half of the sliced green onions. Sauté until aromatic and the onions have softened a bit.
5. Add the soaked and drained noodles to the skillet. Toss them in the oil and aromatics to coat them evenly.
6. Push the noodles to one side of the skillet and pour the beaten egg into the other side. Let it sit for a few moments before scrambling and then mixing it through the noodles.
7. Pour the Pad Thai Sauce over the noodles, stirring to ensure that everything is evenly coated. Cook for a few more minutes until the noodles are tender and the sauce has been absorbed.
8. Add the cooked chicken slices to the skillet, tossing everything together until the chicken is heated through.
9. Squeeze the juice of the lime over the Pad Thai and give it one final toss.
10. Serve the Pad Thai garnished with the remaining green onions, chopped cilantro, and lime wedges on the side.

©Nancy K. Doctor

CONCLUSION

As we wrap up "Diabetic Renal Diet Cookbook For Beginners," let's look back at the adventure we've been on. Starting a new diet might have seemed scary at first, but I hope these recipes and tips have made you feel more confident and excited. This book was made to give you tasty and healthy meal ideas that are perfect for people with diabetes and kidney issues, and to make eating fun again.

Dealing with diabetes and kidney problems can be tough, but having the right information and yummy recipes means you can still enjoy eating while taking good care of yourself. I put a lot of care into creating these recipes, making sure they're just right for your health. I've covered the basics of eating right, like watching your carbs, protein, salt, potassium, and phosphorus, and how being smart about food can make you feel better.

This cookbook isn't just about food; it's a companion to help you on your way to feeling great. The choices you make now can help you feel better later on. I hope the meals you've found here become favorites that make you feel good and happy.

Keep in mind that food is more than just something to eat; it's like a healing tool. It can mend, bring us together, and make happy memories. Let this cookbook remind you that taking care of your health is about living well and finding joy in what you eat.

"Thank you for embarking on this journey with me through this cookbook. Your support inspires hope and empowers change. Together, we navigate the path to wellness, one recipe at a time. Wishing you health, happiness, and delightful culinary adventures."

©Nancy K. Doctor

BONUS

28-Days Meal Plan

Day 1:
- Breakfast: Spicy Tofu Scrambler
- Lunch: Seared Salmon with Braised Broccoli
- Dinner: Gingered Cranberry Chicken Delight
- Snack: Almond Essence Cookies

Day 2:
- Breakfast: Cranberry Almond Bulgur Cereal
- Lunch: Couscous Stuffed Peppers
- Dinner: Zesty Lemon Thyme Tuna Pasta Salad
- Snack: Creamy Peanut Butter Chickpea Dip

Day 3:
- Breakfast: Peanut Butter Infused Oatmeal Bliss
- Lunch: Ultimate Vegetable Stir-Fry
- Dinner: Mexican-Inspired Turkey and Rice Stuffed Peppers
- Snack: Spicy Cream Cheese Tortilla Rolls

Day 4:
- Breakfast: Renal-Friendly Garden Veggie Frittata

- Lunch: Spinach and Mushroom Egg-Light Frittata
- Dinner: Homemade Chicken Pad Thai
- Snack: Strawberry Fruit Salad

Day 5:
- Breakfast: Creamy Peanut Butter Chickpea Dip with whole-grain toast
- Lunch: Herb-Infused French Lentil Salad
- Dinner: Oven-Baked Yogurt and Lemon Chicken Nuggets
- Snack: Almond-Infused Pear Parfait

Day 6:
- Breakfast: Spinach and Mushroom Egg Cups
- Lunch: Sweet Potato Waffles with Homemade Blueberry Syrup
- Dinner: Grilled Pork Tenderloin Fajitas
- Snack: Quick and Nutritious Tuna Salad

Day 7:
- Breakfast: Charred Red Bell Pepper Chickpea Spread on whole-grain toast
- Lunch: Tangy Pickled Onion and Herb Salad
- Dinner: Zesty Fish Tacos with Tomatillo Salsa
- Snack: Nutritious Whole-Grain Soda Bread

Day 8:
- Breakfast: Spicy Tofu Scrambler
- Lunch: Seared Salmon with Braised Broccoli

- Dinner: Gingered Cranberry Chicken Delight
- Snacks: Charred Red Bell Pepper Chickpea Spread; Almond-Infused Pear Parfait

Day 9:
- Breakfast: Renal-Friendly Garden Veggie Frittata
- Lunch: Rosemary Infused Chicken Skewers
- Dinner: Mexican-Inspired Turkey and Rice Stuffed Peppers
- Snacks: Creamy Peanut Butter Chickpea Dip with vegetable sticks; Pear and Fennel Salad with Walnuts

Day 10:
- Breakfast: Cranberry Almond Bulgur Cereal
- Lunch: Oven-Baked Salmon with Asparagus on Whole-Grain Bun
- Dinner: Zesty Lemon Thyme Tuna Pasta Salad
- Snacks: Classic Chickpea Spread with whole-grain crackers; Fresh Spinach and Mixed Berry Salad

Day 11:
- Breakfast: Peanut Butter Infused Oatmeal Bliss
- Lunch: Couscous Stuffed Peppers
- Dinner: Homemade Chicken Pad Thai

- Snacks: Grilled Veggie Avocado Dip with fresh veggies; Honey-Dressed Warm Cabbage and Carrot Slaw

Day 12:
- Breakfast: Spinach and Mushroom Egg Cups
- Lunch: Ultimate Vegetable Stir-Fry
- Dinner: Zesty Fish Tacos with Tomatillo Salsa
- Snacks: Tangy Asparagus Spears; Nutty Chickpea Spread with cucumber slices

Day 13:
- Breakfast: Oven-Baked Yogurt and Lemon Chicken Nuggets
- Lunch: Sweet Potato Waffles with Homemade Blueberry Syrup
- Dinner: Grilled Pork Tenderloin Fajitas
- Snacks: Spinach and Mushroom Egg-Light Frittata; Strawberry Fruit Salad

Day 14:
- Breakfast: Peanut Butter Infused Oatmeal Bliss
- Lunch: Scalloped Corn-Stuffed Bell Peppers
- Dinner: Smoky Bean and Mushroom Cornucopias
- Snacks: Creamy Peanut Butter Chickpea Dip; Chilled Shrimp and Apple Stuffed Tomatoes

Day 15:
- Breakfast: Peanut Butter Infused Oatmeal Bliss
- Lunch: Spring Vegetable Rice Noodles
- Dinner: Gingered Cranberry Chicken Delight
- Snacks: Almond Essence Cookies; Fresh Spinach and Mixed Berry Salad

Day 16:
- Breakfast: Spinach and Mushroom Egg Cups
- Lunch: Sweet Potato Waffles with Homemade Blueberry Syrup
- Dinner: Zesty Lemon Thyme Tuna Pasta Salad
- Snacks: Creamy Greek Yogurt Ranch Dressing with raw veggies; Strawberry Fruit Salad

Day 17 :
- Breakfast: Oven-Baked Yogurt and Lemon Chicken Nuggets
- Lunch: Classic Hummus with vegetable sticks and whole-grain pita
- Dinner: Grilled Pork Tenderloin Fajitas
- Snacks: Cobb Salad with Dijon Dressing; Almond-Infused Pear Parfait

Day 18:
- Breakfast: Cranberry Almond Bulgur Cereal
- Lunch: Tropical Mango Salsa Pizza

- Dinner: Mexican-Inspired Turkey and Rice Stuffed Peppers
- Snacks: Nutritious Tangy Green Beans; Savory Southwestern Cornmeal Muffins

Day 19:
- Breakfast: Spicy Tofu Scrambler
- Lunch: Spinach, Chickpea, and Raisin Pasta
- Dinner: Homemade Chicken Pad Thai
- Snacks: Hearty Vegetable Barley and Mushroom Soup; Berry Delight Whole-Grain Coffee Cake

Day 20:
- Breakfast: Renal-Friendly Garden Veggie Frittata
- Lunch: Smoky Bean and Mushroom Cornucopias
- Dinner: Oven-Baked Salmon with Asparagus on Whole-Grain Bun
- Snacks: Quick Pickled Vegetables; Wholesome Apple Pie (small slice)

Day 21:
- Breakfast: Nutritious Blueberry Whole-Wheat Pancakes
- Lunch: Scalloped Corn-Stuffed Bell Peppers
- Dinner: Rosemary Infused Chicken Skewers
- Snacks: Golden Lemon Almond Rice; Rustic Apple-Cranberry Tart

Day 22:
- Breakfast: Peanut Butter Infused Oatmeal Bliss
- Lunch: Tropical Mango Salsa Pizza
- Dinner: Zesty Lemon Thyme Tuna Pasta Salad
- Snacks: Almond Essence Cookies; Chilled Shrimp and Apple Stuffed Tomatoes

Day 23:
- Breakfast: Oven-Baked Yogurt and Lemon Chicken Nuggets
- Lunch: Smoky Bean and Mushroom Cornucopias
- Dinner: Mexican-Inspired Turkey and Rice Stuffed Peppers
- Snacks: Nutritious Tangy Green Beans; Savory Southwestern Cornmeal Muffins

Day 24:
- Breakfast: Spinach and Mushroom Egg Cups
- Lunch: Spring Vegetable Rice Noodles
- Dinner: Homemade Chicken Pad Thai
- Snacks: Strawberry Fruit Salad; Wholesome Muesli Energy Bars

Day 25:
- Breakfast: Creamy Peanut Butter Chickpea Dip with whole-grain bread
- Lunch: Grilled Pork Tenderloin Fajitas

- Dinner: Gingered Cranberry Chicken Delight
- Snacks: Quick Pickled Vegetables; Berry Delight Whole-Grain Coffee Cake

Day 26:
- Breakfast: Nutritious Whole-Grain Soda Bread with Honeyed Peach Puree
- Lunch: Scalloped Corn-Stuffed Bell Peppers
- Dinner: Seared Salmon with Braised Broccoli
- Snacks: Delicious Spiced Buckwheat Pilaf; Rustic Apple-Cranberry Tart

Day 27:
- Breakfast: Renal-Friendly Garden Veggie Frittata
- Lunch: Zesty Fish Tacos with Tomatillo Salsa
- Dinner: Rosemary Infused Chicken Skewers
- Snacks: Sweet Honey and Sage Glazed Carrots; Warmly Spiced Carrot and Raisin Loaf

Day 28:
- Breakfast: Cranberry Almond Bulgur Cereal
- Lunch: Sweet Potato Waffles with Homemade Blueberry Syrup
- Dinner: Oven-Baked Salmon with Asparagus on Whole-Grain Bun
- Snacks: Tri-Color Tomato Basil Salad; Wholesome Apple Pie

MEAL PLANNER JOURNAL

WEEK: _____ **DATE:** _____

Breakfast _____
Lunch _____
Dinner _____
Snacks _____
Rating your day ○○○○○

Breakfast _____
Lunch _____
Dinner _____
Snacks _____
Rating your day ○○○○○

Breakfast _____
Lunch _____
Dinner _____
Snacks _____
Rating your day ○○○○○

Breakfast _____
Lunch _____
Dinner _____
Snacks _____
Rating your day ○○○○○

Breakfast _____
Lunch _____
Dinner _____
Snacks _____
Rating your day ○○○○○

Breakfast _____
Lunch _____
Dinner _____
Snacks _____
Rating your day ○○○○○

OBSERVATIONS:
_____
_____
_____

MEAL PLANNER JOURNAL

WEEK: _____   **DATE:** _____

| Breakfast |
| Lunch |
| Dinner |
| Snacks |
| Rating your day ○○○○○ |

| Breakfast |
| Lunch |
| Dinner |
| Snacks |
| Rating your day ○○○○○ |

| Breakfast |
| Lunch |
| Dinner |
| Snacks |
| Rating your day ○○○○○ |

| Breakfast |
| Lunch |
| Dinner |
| Snacks |
| Rating your day ○○○○○ |

| Breakfast |
| Lunch |
| Dinner |
| Snacks |
| Rating your day ○○○○○ |

| Breakfast |
| Lunch |
| Dinner |
| Snacks |
| Rating your day ○○○○○ |

| Breakfast |
| Lunch |
| Dinner |
| Snacks |
| Rating your day ○○○○○ |

OBSERVATIONS:

MEAL PLANNER JOURNAL

WEEK: _____   DATE: _____

Breakfast
Lunch
Dinner
Snacks
Rating your day ○○○○○

Breakfast
Lunch
Dinner
Snacks
Rating your day ○○○○○

Breakfast
Lunch
Dinner
Snacks
Rating your day ○○○○○

Breakfast
Lunch
Dinner
Snacks
Rating your day ○○○○○

Breakfast
Lunch
Dinner
Snacks
Rating your day ○○○○○

Breakfast
Lunch
Dinner
Snacks
Rating your day ○○○○○

Breakfast
Lunch
Dinner
Snacks
Rating your day ○○○○○

OBSERVATIONS:

MEAL PLANNER JOURNAL

WEEK: _____ **DATE:** _____

| Breakfast |
| Lunch |
| Dinner |
| Snacks |
| Rating your day ○○○○○ |

| Breakfast |
| Lunch |
| Dinner |
| Snacks |
| Rating your day ○○○○○ |

| Breakfast |
| Lunch |
| Dinner |
| Snacks |
| Rating your day ○○○○○ |

| Breakfast |
| Lunch |
| Dinner |
| Snacks |
| Rating your day ○○○○○ |

| Breakfast |
| Lunch |
| Dinner |
| Snacks |
| Rating your day ○○○○○ |

| Breakfast |
| Lunch |
| Dinner |
| Snacks |
| Rating your day ○○○○○ |

| Breakfast |
| Lunch |
| Dinner |
| Snacks |
| Rating your day ○○○○○ |

OBSERVATIONS:

MEAL PLANNER JOURNAL

WEEK: _____   DATE: _____

Breakfast _____
Lunch _____
Dinner _____
Snacks _____
Rating your day ○○○○○

Breakfast _____
Lunch _____
Dinner _____
Snacks _____
Rating your day ○○○○○

Breakfast _____
Lunch _____
Dinner _____
Snacks _____
Rating your day ○○○○○

Breakfast _____
Lunch _____
Dinner _____
Snacks _____
Rating your day ○○○○○

Breakfast _____
Lunch _____
Dinner _____
Snacks _____
Rating your day ○○○○○

Breakfast _____
Lunch _____
Dinner _____
Snacks _____
Rating your day ○○○○○

Breakfast _____
Lunch _____
Dinner _____
Snacks _____
Rating your day ○○○○○

OBSERVATIONS:
_____
_____
_____
_____

MEAL PLANNER JOURNAL

WEEK: _____ **DATE:** _____

| Breakfast _____ |
| Lunch _____ |
| Dinner _____ |
| Snacks _____ |
| Rating your day ○○○○○ |

| Breakfast _____ |
| Lunch _____ |
| Dinner _____ |
| Snacks _____ |
| Rating your day ○○○○○ |

| Breakfast _____ |
| Lunch _____ |
| Dinner _____ |
| Snacks _____ |
| Rating your day ○○○○○ |

| Breakfast _____ |
| Lunch _____ |
| Dinner _____ |
| Snacks _____ |
| Rating your day ○○○○○ |

| Breakfast _____ |
| Lunch _____ |
| Dinner _____ |
| Snacks _____ |
| Rating your day ○○○○○ |

| Breakfast _____ |
| Lunch _____ |
| Dinner _____ |
| Snacks _____ |
| Rating your day ○○○○○ |

| Breakfast _____ |
| Lunch _____ |
| Dinner _____ |
| Snacks _____ |
| Rating your day ○○○○○ |

OBSERVATIONS:
_____
_____
_____
_____

MEAL PLANNER JOURNAL

WEEK: _____   **DATE:** _____

Breakfast _____
Lunch _____
Dinner _____
Snacks _____

Rating your day ○○○○○

Breakfast _____
Lunch _____
Dinner _____
Snacks _____

Rating your day ○○○○○

Breakfast _____
Lunch _____
Dinner _____
Snacks _____

Rating your day ○○○○○

Breakfast _____
Lunch _____
Dinner _____
Snacks _____

Rating your day ○○○○○

Breakfast _____
Lunch _____
Dinner _____
Snacks _____

Rating your day ○○○○○

Breakfast _____
Lunch _____
Dinner _____
Snacks _____

Rating your day ○○○○○

Breakfast _____
Lunch _____
Dinner _____
Snacks _____

Rating your day ○○○○○

OBSERVATIONS:
_____
_____
_____
_____

©Nancy K. Doctor

MEAL PLANNER JOURNAL

WEEK: _____   DATE: _____

Breakfast _____
Lunch _____
Dinner _____
Snacks _____
Rating your day ○ ○ ○ ○ ○

Breakfast _____
Lunch _____
Dinner _____
Snacks _____
Rating your day ○ ○ ○ ○ ○

Breakfast _____
Lunch _____
Dinner _____
Snacks _____
Rating your day ○ ○ ○ ○ ○

Breakfast _____
Lunch _____
Dinner _____
Snacks _____
Rating your day ○ ○ ○ ○ ○

Breakfast _____
Lunch _____
Dinner _____
Snacks _____
Rating your day ○ ○ ○ ○ ○

Breakfast _____
Lunch _____
Dinner _____
Snacks _____
Rating your day ○ ○ ○ ○ ○

Breakfast _____
Lunch _____
Dinner _____
Snacks _____
Rating your day ○ ○ ○ ○ ○

OBSERVATIONS:
_____
_____
_____
_____

©Nancy K. Doctor

Groceries Shopping List Planner

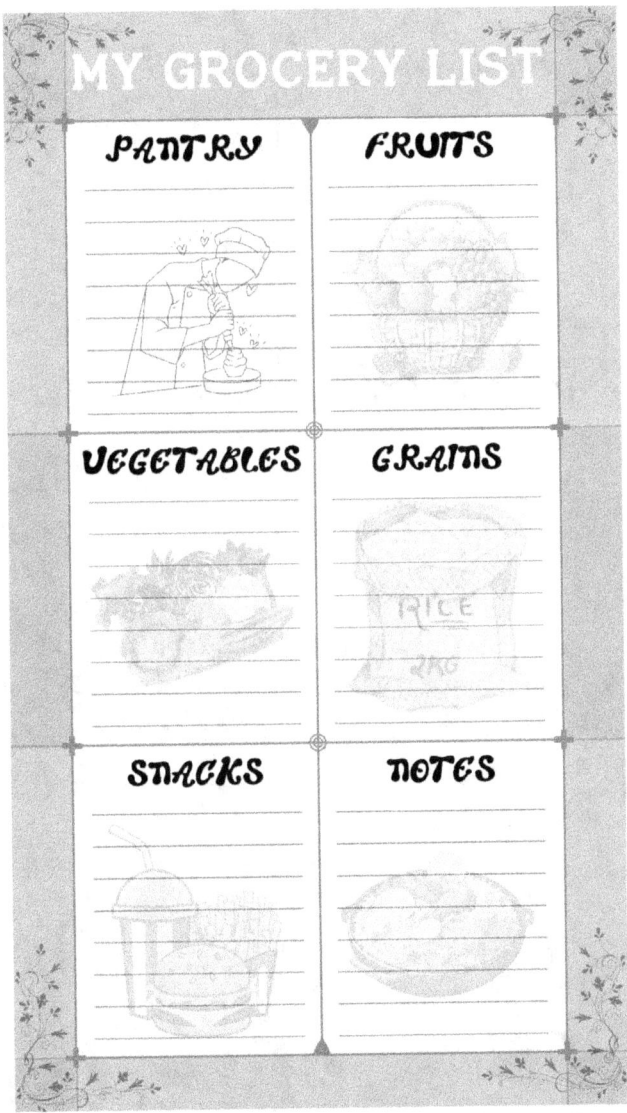

MY GROCERY LIST

PANTRY

FRUITS

VEGETABLES

GRAINS

SNACKS

NOTES

©Nancy K. Doctor

MY GROCERY LIST

PANTRY	FRUITS

VEGETABLES	GRAINS

SNACKS	NOTES

MY GROCERY LIST

PANTRY

FRUITS

VEGETABLES

GRAINS

SNACKS

NOTES

©Nancy K. Doctor

MY GROCERY LIST

PANTRY

FRUITS

VEGETABLES

GRAINS

SNACKS

NOTES

DIABETIC RENAL DIET COOKBOOK FOR BEGINNERS

©Nancy K. Doctor

MY GROCERY LIST

PANTRY	FRUITS
VEGETABLES	GRAINS
SNACKS	NOTES

DIABETIC RENAL DIET COOKBOOK FOR BEGINNERS

©Nancy K. Doctor

MY GROCERY LIST

PANTRY

FRUITS

VEGETABLES

GRAINS

SNACKS

NOTES

©Nancy K. Doctor

MY GROCERY LIST

PANTRY

FRUITS

VEGETABLES

GRAINS

SNACKS

NOTES

DIABETIC RENAL DIET COOKBOOK FOR BEGINNERS

©Nancy K. Doctor

The Free Ebook Download

Scan the QR Code With your Phone to Download the Free Ebook Version of This Book ⬇

©Nancy K. Doctor

OTHER BOOKS WRITTEN BY THE AUTHOR

Scan the QR Code below the image of Any of the Books 👇

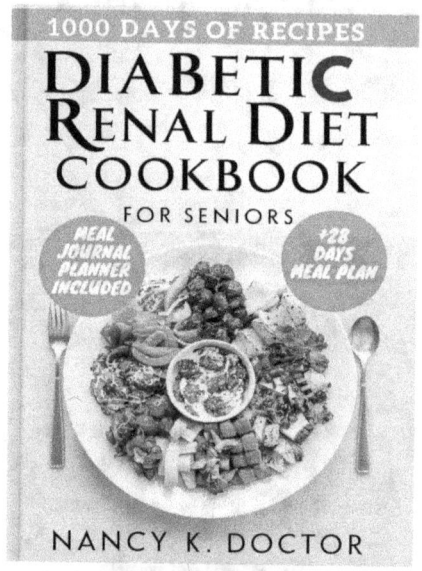

©Nancy K. Doctor

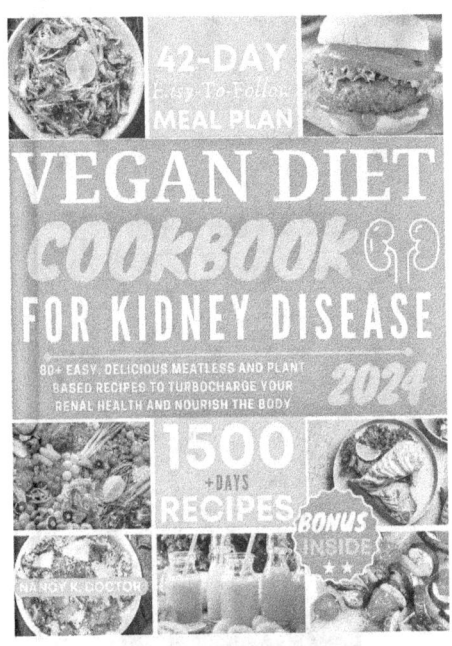

Vegan Renal Diet

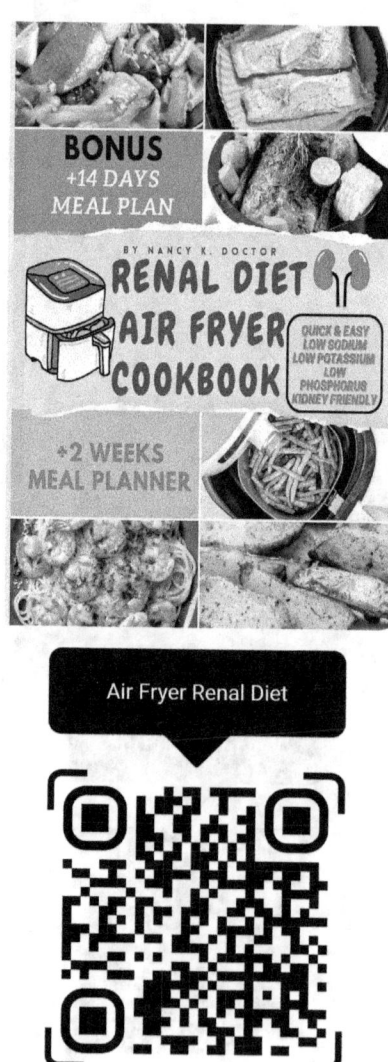

©Nancy K. Doctor

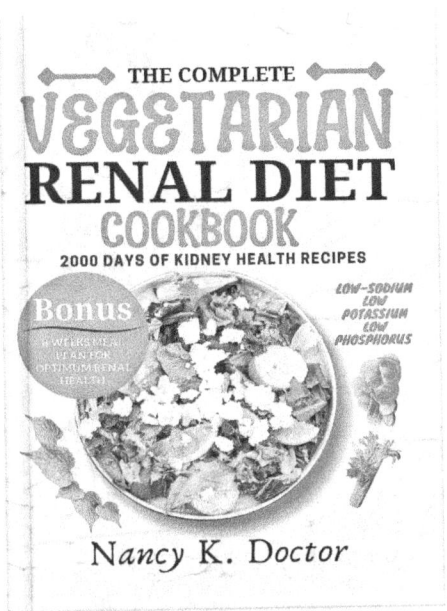

©Nancy K. Doctor

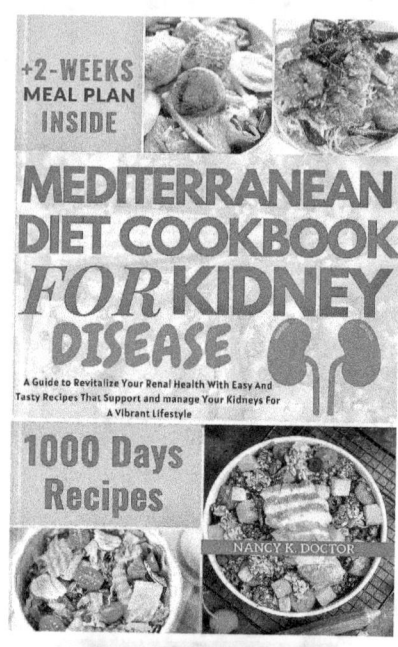

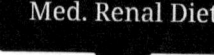

©Nancy K. Doctor

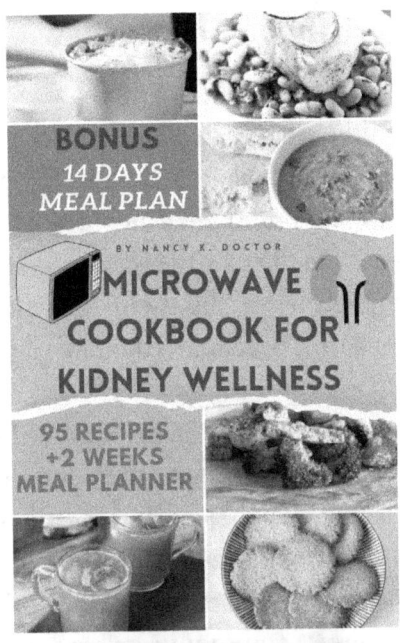

Microwave Renal Diet

©Nancy K. Doctor

About The Author

Dr. Nancy K. Doctor, a passionate advocate for kidney health, has dedicated her career to empowering individuals affected by kidney disease and diabetes. As a renowned nephrologist, certified dietician, and seasoned fitness coach, she brings a unique perspective to the field, merging medical knowledge with practical dietary and lifestyle solutions.

For over two decades, Dr. Nancy has guided countless patients through the complexities of kidney disease & Diabetes, helping them navigate dietary limitations and embrace healthier living. Her commitment extends beyond the clinic, as she actively inspires communities through lectures, workshops, and her bestselling books, "Renal Diet Cookbook For Seniors: A Holistic Guide to Recovery and Resilience through Dieting."

Driven by a belief that delicious food and empowered choices can pave the way to renal well-being, Dr. Nancy is always on the lookout for innovative approaches. Witnessing the potential of air fryer technology to create exciting and flavorful kidney-friendly dishes spurred her latest project, "Diabetic Renal Diet Cookbook For Beginners."

This book, though just one facet of Dr. Nancy's multifaceted contribution to kidney health and Diabetes, exemplifies her unwavering dedication to making delicious, nutritious food accessible for everyone on their renal journey. Whether through Snacks, Smoothies, Microwave, air fryer magic or other empowering resources, Dr. Nancy remains a beacon of hope, guiding individuals towards a healthier, happier life with kidney disease and Diabetes.

To learn more About the Author and other books written by her; Scan the QR Code below

www.ingramcontent.com/pod-product-compliance
Lightning Source LLC
Chambersburg PA
CBHW052202220526
45471CB00004B/1776